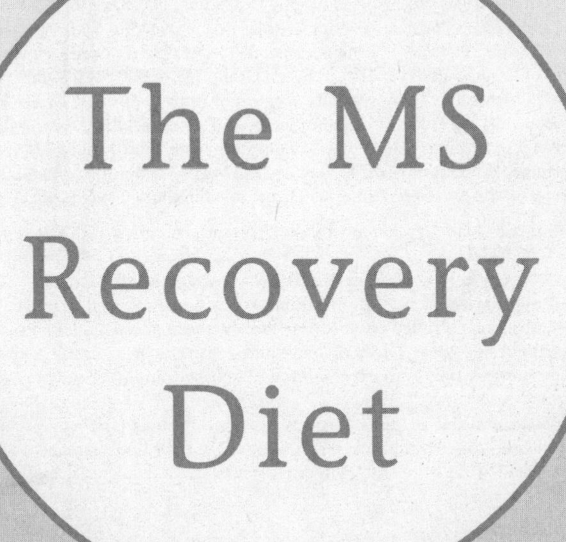

The MS Recovery Diet

Take Control, Change What You Eat, and Live Symptom-Free

Ann D. Sawyer
and Judith E. Bachrach

Published by the Penguin Group
Penguin Group (USA) Inc., 375 Hudson Street, New York, New York 10014, USA • Penguin Group (Canada), 90 Eglinton Avenue East, Suite 700, Toronto, Ontario M4P 2Y3, Canada (a division of Pearson Penguin Canada Inc.) • Penguin Books Ltd, 80 Strand, London WC2R 0RL, England • Penguin Ireland, 25 St Stephen's Green, Dublin 2, Ireland (a division of Penguin Books Ltd) • Penguin Group (Australia), 250 Camberwell Road, Camberwell, Victoria 3124, Australia (a division of Pearson Australia Group Pty Ltd) • Penguin Books India Pvt Ltd, 11 Community Centre, Panchsheel Park, New Delhi–110 017, India • Penguin Group (NZ), 67 Apollo Drive, Rosedale, North Shore 0745, Auckland, New Zealand (a division of Pearson New Zealand Ltd) • Penguin Books (South Africa) (Pty) Ltd, 24 Sturdee Avenue, Rosebank, Johannesburg 2196, South Africa

Penguin Books Ltd, Registered Offices: 80 Strand, London WC2R 0RL, England

ISBN 978-1-58333-288-7

Printed in the United States of America
13 15 17 19 20 18 16 14 12

BOOK DESIGN BY NICOLE LAROCHE

To all the indomitable pioneers of diet and nutritional treatment for MS who refused to accept the one-way journey to disability, and instead blazed the healing trail for the rest of us to follow.

I'm flying on the wings of heaven
I'm growing from the roots of earth
I'm burning with the fire of light
I'm carried on the river of life

—From Judi's song
"Flying on the Wings of Heaven"

Ann's Acknowledgments

This book, several years in the making, bears the imprint of many people to whom I owe a debt of gratitude.

My husband Steve's voice was the strongest in urging me to take on this project, so without him there would be no book. Throughout, he has been totally supportive in so many ways, including editing and straightening out my messes on the computer. He is my rock.

I am grateful to all the people who've beaten MS and then shared their knowledge and experience. A special thanks to Ashton Embry for all his work in gathering the scientific information, followed by consolidating the MS Recovery Diet. He has been tireless in reaching out to help others by disseminating this treatment information. More personally, I thank him for his support of my writing this book.

In my personal life, I can't say enough about the love, caring, and support I received from my children, Kate, Andrew, and Edward, through my whole MS odyssey. My friends, too, were always there for me as they witnessed my fight against MS. This fine group includes: Cindie Aadland, Joretta Barbee, Jean Braithwaite, Nora Brashear, Stef

Breslin, Lisa Kilburg, Martha Lindquist, Barb Patschke, Meg Strohmer, and Barbara Tabbert.

Many thanks to Darlene, Ruth, Carol, Letia, and Bryon for generously sharing their MS stories, which are included in this book. And to my readers, who offered invaluable suggestions: Laura Derr, Laurie Shelton, Arlene Uslander, and Laura Fendt.

I am grateful to have found Judi. I needed someone to help write a cookbook and compile information about exercise. This is the offer I made to her: "We may never publish, but we can print the books ourselves and give them out to those who need them"—as I had been doing for several years. With no prospect of gain, beyond the satisfaction of truly helping to relieve suffering, Judi signed on and has put her heart and soul into this book.

The Avery imprint of the Penguin Group will forever have my respect for the courage shown in publishing this book. Megan Newman, the publisher, and Lucia Watson, the senior editor, have been totally supportive in helping us to polish and refine our manuscript.

Judi's Acknowledgments

Thank you to my beloved husband, Richard. Your unending love, patience, and support have sustained me through what otherwise seemed unbearable. For this project, you have been First Sounding Board, First Reader, First Editor, and First Fan. My love and gratitude to you, always and forever.

To my daughters, Emilia and Marion, I give thanks for seeing me beyond the ill mother I was for so many years and into my recovery and for your enthusiastic endorsement of the creation of this book. You are the best, most honest, and loving life partners anyone could ever have.

Ann, you have my gratitude for being a new friend and partner. You are a woman of intelligence and conviction who invited me to co-create my bridge to health through the information and creation of this book. The crossing of our paths is no coincidence, and I still see a long, straight road before us as ambassadors of this message. I also am thankful for the constructive criticism from your daughter, Kate, and for all the time and clear eye for detail brought to this project by your husband, Steve.

Thanks also to the clients, students, and strangers with MS who have chosen to share their personal journeys with me.

I want to thank my extended family and also my many friends both here and abroad who have kept me in their hearts and prayers for years. I can mention only a few of you who were also involved with my recovery: Howard Bornstein for your tech support, business advice, photographic skills, healing heart, and healing hands (Feldenkrais, NSR, and jin shin jyustu), and for your wife, Kathy Vian, for her many gifts, among them great cooking. I thank my longtime friends and fellow spiritual seekers: Len and Ellen Holmes, for sharing our abundant life gardens; Phyllis Luberg, for mothering everything with me; and Kim Rosen, for being the brilliant, creative wordsmith that you are. My gratitude to Geoffrey Kuhrts for several of your recipes, and to Dennis and Carol McCarthey, Einer and Natalie Mortensen, and the many of you unmentioned. I thank you all for the opportunity to cook and share many healthy feasts of delight.

Naming the number of healers I have worked with throughout the years would require an entire book, so I can only say thank you from my heart to yours for your gifts and wisdom. I thank here my current Pilates instructor and Shiatsu practitioner, Maiya Greaves, whose exercise ideas supporting my recovery can be found in this book (though all mistakes or confusing language are mine and mine alone), and her profound connection to Unci Maka, which can be found in the world around us. I also thank Mette Coleman, my physical therapist, who has the best osteopathic approach I know, and who can articulate and track every triumph of recovery I have made—and have yet to make—with her skillful and compassionate help. I arrived here through my previous years of work with Bert Shaw, Emilie Conrad, Susan Harper, Jason and Arlene Shulman, Barbara Brennan, and so many others.

I want to thank Megan Newman, publisher at Avery, for recognizing the much-needed hope and truth in our first rough manuscript; Lucia Watson, senior editor at Avery, for her delightful and very skilled midwifery of all versions of this book; and all of the supporting people at Avery for helping us deliver this book to relieve the suffering of so many.

Contents

PART 2

Stories of Healing

PART 3

The MS Recovery Diet Cookbook

Introduction: Two MS Worlds

I love the wild parts of Hawaii, where nature shows her splendor and man's presence is barely felt. On a recent visit to Maui, my husband and I hiked down a cinder trail into the moonscape crater of the Haleakala volcano, up the Napili coast, down the beaches extending south from it, and on Kauai, into the Waimea Canyon, which is two-thirds the size of the Grand Canyon. It was a glorious trip, made all the more miraculous because I have multiple sclerosis.

MS is defined as a demyelinating and degenerative disease of the central nervous system in which the fatty, insulating sheath around the nerves—the myelin—is damaged or destroyed by inflammatory action. In a second, related disease pathway, recently identified and not well understood, the axons, which are the long fibers of the nerve, are destroyed within normal-looking white and gray matter. This second process is the primary source of disability. It was previously thought that disability was caused by lesions on the spinal cord or brain. Both the lesions (or sclerosis or plaques) and the axonal destruction interfere with the conduction of nerve impulses. This disruption of nerve conduction results in a loss of function that may include visual problems,

problems with walking, numbness, weakness, fatigue, and a whole array of other symptoms that usually worsen over time. But I have found that this does not have to be the case; MS can be controlled and reversed.

Welcome to an MS world that is not dark and dismal, but a place filled with hope, progress, and gratitude. Those of us who have found the way to control and reverse our symptoms talk about the new discoveries each of us has made in solving our individual MS puzzle. We swap recipes and tell humorous stories of our misadventures. The people who populate my MS world have not only stopped the disease progression, but actually reversed it, by healing and restoring their abilities. We look to the future with the expectation of health, and we've done that with nothing more than making specific changes in our diet. We haven't found a wonder drug or engaged in potentially dangerous treatment protocols, and we certainly haven't done it by using the medications that are usually prescribed to MS sufferers.

At most, our MS is now a minor inconvenience, and we are confident in our ability to heal and to keep the disease under control. Strange as it may seem, most of us are grateful for our MS, for it has taught us valuable lessons, helped us to grow, and guided us to a new, more empowered place in our lives.

Contrast ours to the MS world of allopathic medicine and the National Multiple Sclerosis Society (NMSS), where progress is defined as the slowing of the progressive downward spiral into disability. By their understanding, after the disease has developed to secondary progressive and symptoms remain constant, there is permanent damage and scarring, which can't be reversed, and abilities lost, which can't be restored. NMSS literature focuses on the best medications to help manage symptoms, showcases wheelchairs and other health aids, and offers advice on how to talk to your doctor. Scientific journal articles describe the irreversible nerve damage done by MS. They cite new drugs on the horizon that really promise no more than do the current offerings designed to slow the progression of the disease. The literature makes valiant efforts to put a happy face on the MS world by featuring people who have made the best of life despite their handicaps, but those articles usually fall short. The MS world of conventional medicine does not include any promise of recovery or control; indeed, it has delivered only spotty results in stopping the progression.

I can't resolve these two MS worlds. It is the exact same disease in all of us. We all have the clinical markers—namely, the lesions on our central nervous system as seen in an MRI; the oligoclonal band, showing the presence of discrete immunoglobulin cells (IgA, IgG, for instance) in the cerebrospinal fluid, indicating immune system activity within the central nervous system; MBP (myelin basic protein), the myelin breakdown product in our spinal fluid; abnormal evoke potentials (tests that measure the location and extent of decreased electrical conduction by our nerves)—and we all have similar clinical histories. Some of us who have recovered had advanced MS for long periods of time, so it isn't that we've had milder cases. We have all been officially diagnosed by the medical establishment.

I am not going to try to explain the vast differences between these two MS worlds. Rather, I am going to present our world with the hope that it will be a healing guide for others with multiple sclerosis. Personally, I am filled with gratitude for having been shown this path. It gave me entrance to wild Hawaii and an unrestricted life. I was lucky to find this information and to tap into a network of people who had recovered from MS, and that has made all the difference in my life.

The Birth of *The MS Recovery Diet*

Initially, I resisted writing this book. "My story isn't sufficiently interesting," I thought. "Besides, I don't want to make a career of MS. It is simply not on my mind anymore." My passion for the topic was fading along with my symptoms.

Ultimately, however, what compelled me to write *The MS Recovery Diet* was the opportunity to pass on the keys to healing that I was so generously given by others to help in my own recovery. I am not a heroine in this story. I did nothing original and made no discoveries. I am just a very thankful recipient of information that has been helping people with MS to recover for more than fifty years.

The true heroes of my story are Dr. Roy Swank, who for forty years studied and treated MS patients through diet modification; Roger MacDougall, who discovered the way to recover from his own debilitating MS; Judy Graham, who recovered many of her lost abilities and then wrote about her success for others to read; and Ashton Embry, who continues to gather and disseminate scientific papers supporting the legitimacy of the Recovery Diet and who lobbies to get it accepted into mainstream medicine. These individuals all had the courage to go against the authority and pronouncements of the medical establishment. And they had the generosity of heart to share their knowledge through whatever means were available—in books and articles, on the Internet, and through word of mouth. If it weren't for these pioneers and all the other people who recovered and added to this growing body of knowledge, this program of treatment would not have been developed. I am also grateful that it was available to me and to those whose stories I tell and the many others who have used it. Without the efforts of so many who contributed pieces of knowledge about healing, our stories would have taken a much different and sadder turn. How, then, could I not do my best to contribute by collating this information and writing this book?

It may seem presumptuous to advocate the effectiveness of something as simple as a change in diet when the best minds of medicine have come up with little more than palliatives and Band-Aids. But no matter how much doubt the establishment casts upon the diet/nutritional treatment approach, the fact remains that it has worked for many people who were willing to take the challenge.

There is no known cure for the disease; however, the Recovery Diet works to reverse and control its symptoms. When followed conscientiously, it restores normal functioning so that MS becomes not the defining force of one's everyday life, but an incidental and inconsequential medical diagnosis. No other treatment can make this claim. The need for an absolute cure fades when MS is reduced to a footnote by your name.

I was lucky to find the right book in the bookstore, to come across the right essay on the Internet, to know someone who knew someone who had recovered from MS through the Recovery Diet. I hope this book will be the lucky talisman for you or someone you know to forge a unique healing path from the scourge of MS.

More recently, I was fortunate in meeting Judi, who not only is further validating the diet by her remarkable recovery from very progressed MS but also has the talent and interest to help me fill out this book, especially with her contributions to the cookbook section.

We can't in good conscience advocate that anyone use this diet as a substitute for good medical advice and care, but we urge you to give it a chance. There are no risks, only benefits to be had. And, if it works for you, as we think it will, please pass it on.

The MS Recovery Diet

This book is a complete guide to healing from MS, meaning that symptoms will be eliminated, or at least be reduced to a minor inconvenience. Judi and I intend that it be easy to use this book as a reference guide. We have arranged the chapters so that you can go back to certain sections time and again. Each chapter is also self-contained, should you want to skip around, although we encourage cover-to-cover reading initially.

The book is divided into the following four sections:

Part 1 reviews what MS is, using the latest research, and then outlines the specifics of the diet and why it works. Since the program is the reason any reader picks up this book, we go right to this first but then continue to document and supply more information in the following chapters. The history of MS places the dietary approach in context, and traces its development. In addressing the accompanying difficulties of

MS, we illuminate the darkness of depression and suggest different ways to handle it. No matter how physically compromised the reader may be, we explain the importance of exercise and give clear written instructions of how to begin this dynamic aspect of recovery. We offer suggestions for the best ways to maintain your recovery, emphasizing the positives of this new lifestyle. Embarking on this diet affects every aspect of your life: acquiring a new view of food, from how you cook to going out to eat; coping with changing expectations on all sides; your relationship to your body; how you see yourself as you emerge from MS's grip, to name a few. We try to address these issues not only in a short conclusion at the end of this section but also throughout the book.

Part 2 offers the reader our own MS stories, as well as those of other men and women who have recovered from the disease. These profiles were carefully selected to show how each case is unique, just as is each person's experience of the disease. As you see how others solved their puzzles, we hope you will gain insights for your own healing journey.

Part 3 gets down to the business of food. For someone with MS, food has the power to hurt as well as to heal. Even more than for the average person, food is essential to our health and sense of well-being. Knowing how hard it can be to make the changes necessary to healing, we present a full cookbook offering ways of eating to satisfy all lifestyles. Even for the noncook, the range of recipes and suggestions makes following the diet easier. The extensive recipe section is both for those who like to cook and those who wonder if they will ever again be able to eat a beloved comfort food. We are pleased to say those dishes are not lost forever; there are recipes using substitutions that reproduce your favorites. Beyond the recipes, this cookbook gives sample menus and shows how to follow the diet and make good food choices at home or dining out.

The last part of the book includes a bibliography and three appendixes, which contain an extensive list of supplements that can augment the program, a list of resources such as bodywork and exercise formats, and a review of other alternative healing modalities.

We wish you the best of luck on your healing journey and hope that you find the same success that we have with the MS Recovery Diet.

PART 1

The MS Recovery Diet

1

What Is MS?

Multiple sclerosis (MS) is a disease in which central nervous system (CNS) damage results in compromised electrical conduction in the nerves. The lack of or poor nerve signals can result in minor annoyances or total disability. These symptoms include altered sensations, impaired vision, loss of muscle coordination, incontinence, and cognitive problems in thinking and memory, just to name a few. The disease course is variable and unpredictable, but usually it starts slowly with periodic eruptions between apparent times of normalcy before progressing to being fully active with permanent, often debilitating symptoms. As a result, more than three-quarters of the people affected have some disability or limitation, and one-quarter become wheelchair-bound.

This definition barely begins to describe MS, for it is a complex and perplexing disease that has, so far, baffled science and thwarted any true understanding. "Multiple" is the word that best describes this disease; it has multiple predisposing factors, multiple disease pathways, multiple symptoms, and involves multiple body systems. In sum, this disease continues to raise multiple questions.

Much of what is known about MS is merely descriptive—science has not progressed to the point that all the known facts can be placed into a context of understanding. A good way to explain MS, for the purposes of this book, is to follow the experiences of MS from first manifestation through diagnosis and to the end prognosis.

Basic Facts About MS

MS gets its name from the hardened white tissue found around the areas of destruction in the brain or on the spinal cord, where the disruption of the electrical messages of the nerves occurs. These hardened tissue areas are also called scars, sclerosis, plaques, or lesions. These can be seen on MRIs and have been thought to be the hallmark of MS.

Myelin, the insulating fatty sheath surrounding the nerves, is the focus for this destruction. Various cells, both the attackers and those sent to clean up the site, constitute the lesions where the myelin has been destroyed.

Recently, a second disease path has been articulated in which the nerve axons, the long fibers of the nerve cells that act like fiber-optic cords, are destroyed. This pathway is primarily responsible for the resulting disability, but had remained undetected because this destruction occurs under normal-appearing white matter and gray matter. The white matter is those nerve cells that are myelinated, getting their designation from white coloration. The nerve cells in the cortex of the brain are more densely packed and not myelinated, and therefore appear gray. This is a new development, for MS historically was only considered to affect the white matter, specifically in attacks on the myelin.

Over its history, MS has been referred to as a vascular disease, an infectious disease, a genetic disease, an environmental disease, an allergic disease, an inflammatory disease, and an autoimmune disease. There is evidence for each case. An autoimmune disease is defined as being related to or caused by the body's specialized immune cells designed to attack outside antigens (foreign bodies) which instead attack the self cells. Though MS doesn't have definitive autoimmune markers, there is strong evidence for autoimmune activity, such as the presence of IgG (immunoglobulin G, which shows antibody formation), which is found within the OB (oligoclonal band, an indication of antibodies) in the spinal fluid of the CNS.

A vascular disease relates to the circulatory systems, specifically the blood vessels in the case of MS. Breaches in the microscopic capillaries next to the spinal cord allow immune cells to cross what should be an impenetrable blood-brain barrier into the CNS.

The First Introduction—Symptoms

A brief spell of blurry vision, a tightness or numbness in the legs, or an electric shock racing down your spine is often the first calling card of MS. Even before that, you may have had a vague feeling that something was not quite right with you, a greater sensitivity to heat or cold, or several unexplained bruises. No one could ever have identified these events as MS, but the disease was already stirring. Out of sight and undetected, these first subtle markers can easily be dismissed. Fatigue, unlike any you have ever known before, may also appear, only to be explained away by modern life.

Visual problems, like blind spots or a dimming or blurring of images, and sensory problems, such as weakness, pins and needles, or numbness, are the most common initial symptoms, but MS can potentially affect any body part or function. It can often be first identified by the rapid onset of symptoms, which can last seconds, minutes, hours, weeks, or years.

Over the course of the disease, you develop a unique symptom profile as the same strange happenings reappear during the relapsing and remitting stage of the disease, only to become permanent as the disease progresses. Some studies suggest that, on average, any one person will only experience six or seven different symptoms throughout their lives.

It is important to know what symptoms are characteristic of MS, both to be able to gauge your disease activity as well as to differentiate health problems unrelated to MS. It is too easy to attribute every odd sensation and feeling to this enigmatic disease and miss treating some other health issue. Though the symptoms are placed in a category to reflect the kind of problem—cerebellar for brain, sensory for sensation, motor for movement—you will notice that, like everything else about MS, it is not so simple and there are overlaps and multiple category involvement. Here is a list of the MS symptoms:

Fatigue

This is by far the most common and most misunderstood of all symptoms. "Fatigue" is a common word denoting a common experience shared by everyone; however, the word doesn't truly describe the totally overwhelming and paralyzing symptom of MS. "Multisystem failure" more accurately captures what happens when all physical, emotional, and cognitive functioning shuts down with the total depletion of any energy available. You could drop things, fall down, stumble or be dizzy, be unable to think or remember or even talk clearly, or shed tears of unexplained anger or frustration for no apparent reason. With all this, you would have an urgent need to lie down because there is nothing else you can do. That is multisystem failure, usually referred to as MS fatigue.

Sensory and Motor Symptoms

Specific symptoms do not correlate to the location of the lesions, nor does the size of the lesion indicate the severity of the symptom. Little is understood about why a particular symptom appears in one person and not another. However, lesions do correlate to the breaches in the blood-brain barrier.

PARESTHESIA—Altered sensations that can affect any part of the body include numbness, tingling, feeling hot or cold, a painful burning sensation, or tightness or banding, usually around the torso. Creepy-crawly sensations anywhere on the body may also occur.

A paralysis of the facial nerve, temporary or permanent, may occur, usually on one side of the face; this facial paralysis is known as Bell's palsy.

A sensation of an electric shock going down the spinal cord and out the limbs when the head is bowed is known as Lhermitte's sign.

SPASTICITY—A limb or muscle becomes tight and stiff because of spontaneous contraction and resists any relaxation. This may manifest as clonus, an involuntary jerking of the leg due to repeated spastic contractions; extension spasm, whereby the leg freezes in an extended position and will not bend; or flexor spasm, where the leg freezes in fetal position. Each of these can be very painful.

WEAKNESS—A muscle or limb can give out inexplicably, making people fall or drop whatever they are holding. People prone to this symptom are often afraid to walk or hold things, as they never know when this symptom will strike. When this weakness affects one side of the body, the condition is known as hemiparesis.

TREMORS—Uncontrollable shaking can occur. Intentional tremor, one of the first symptoms identified, refers to the shaking of the hand when there is purposeful movement. A tremor of the neck and head is known as titubation.

PARALYSIS—Paralysis in some or all of the muscles can occur. Hemiplegia, the paralysis of one side of the body, is also a symptom.

BLADDER AND BOWEL DYSFUNCTION—Symptoms can vary from inability to release to loss of control.

ATAXIA—Poor coordination resulting in difficulty in doing a simple physical task, due to lack of muscular control or proper nerve messages.

Again, there are specific conditions such as dysmetria, in which a person overreaches an object, or stance ataxia, which is the inability to stand. These are also cerebellar symptoms.

Cerebellar Symptoms

VERTIGO—This is a feeling of dizziness or spinning, which results in problems of balance or even the inability to sit or stand.

COGNITIVE DYSFUNCTION—All mental functions, including memory, word retrieval, decision making, the ordering of thoughts, and retention of knowledge, can be compromised by MS. Research shows that more than half of all MS cases have such difficulties.

EMOTIONAL PROBLEMS—The emotions can be affected with increased lability, the person swinging between extreme feelings, as well as expressing inappropriate affect, like laughing when there is nothing funny. People with MS also are more vulnerable to clinical depression.

HEADACHES—Headaches can appear in any quadrant, including just one side of the head or the other.

VISUAL PROBLEMS—Such abnormalities can include diplopia, or double vision; nystagmus, or rapid involuntary movement of the eyeballs, usually horizontally; and scotoma, or having a blind spot. With enough damage to the optic nerve, blindness can result.

SPEECH PROBLEMS—Disorders can range from dysarthria, or poorly articulated words, to dysphonia, or poor tonal quality.

HEARING PROBLEMS—Again, hearing is also dependent on the nerves to function and carry messages, so such impairment with MS is common.

HEAT—Both the heat of the sun and air as well as heat from water can cause extreme weakness or failure of the muscles, but other symptoms may manifest. It is thought that heat limits conduction, so the solution is to cool off and often the previous level of function is restored.

PAIN—Though the manifestation of neurologically caused pain is not understood, it is a very real symptom and can affect any part of the body.

Late-Appearing Symptoms

These appear at the end of the disease, and include trouble swallowing and breathing, as well as a paralysis that resembles a stroke.

Diagnosis

At some point, a person experiencing symptoms for a long period of time or a person suffering from an acute symptom will consult a health-care professional. More often, they will see several medical people over a period of time, and for good reason. MS is hard to diagnose conclusively.

Reasons for this difficulty: most of the MS symptoms are also found in other diseases, and clinical measures are not unique to MS. Ever elusive, the first symptoms that manifest in MS are usually transient and can be vague, like a generalized strange feeling that leaves no evidence on which to make a diagnosis. Even if the symptoms remain, there is no definitive marker for MS.

The diagnosis is most often made through the process of elimination and by evidence of the end-point damage. The usual procedure is to eliminate other more definitive diseases, such as Lyme disease, brain tumors, pinched nerves and slipped disks, diabetic neuritis, thyroid disease, psychological problems, reaction to medications, peripheral neuralgia, and vitamin B deficiency, to name a few possibilities. A diagnosis requires at least two attacks, involving some of the symptoms listed above.

The medical tests used for diagnosis are MRI scans, a spinal tap, and evoked potential tests. All can be useful, but they have their drawbacks.

The MRI, or magnetic resonance imager, provides a picture of the spinal cord and brain. Lesions show up as shadowy white or gray patches on the film, which make reading them an art as much as a science. Other diseases can cause such patches, as does the process of aging, so these are more useful to confirm, rather than to establish, MS. There is weak correlation between the patches seen on the MRI and clinical signs.

In recent years, with better imaging and clinical technology, a second disease path has been discovered, which is now understood to be the primary mechanism that leads to disability. This axonal damage that occurs under normal-appearing white or gray matter is not detected by traditional MRI imaging. Because the correlation between the lesions that do appear in the films and this axonal damage is not definitive, true diagnosis and evaluation of disease activity is more limited than originally thought with the MRI.

In a spinal tap, a needle is inserted into the intrathecal space, the area surrounding the brain and spinal cord that holds the cerebrospinal fluid. A sample of the fluid is drawn for analysis. This is a highly sensitive area, so the procedure presents a risk of infection and problems, like headaches and dizziness. The presence of IgG or OB in the fluid suggests the presence of autoimmune activity. A finding of MBP (myelin basic protein) indicates the breakdown of myelin. These findings are not unique to MS, however, and MS can also exist without leaving these telltale signs.

The evoked potential test measures the electrical response to stimulation along the nerve pathways, noting the locations of loss of conduction. These are run from the eyes to the brain, and the fingers and toes to the brain, with electrodes along the pathway. This test can differentiate whether the problem is in the CNS or in the peripheral nerves. But again, other diseases, such as lupus and neurosyphilis, may have similar results on this test indicating CNS involvement.

There are no absolutes in diagnosing MS. A person can have the disease without leaving any fingerprints that show up on any of the tests. And again, the diagnosis only describes the end point or manifestation of the disease process. Unlike many other diseases, MS has no specific virus, genetic marker, chemical marker in the blood system, or anything that relates to the disease's cause to make a firm diagnosis.

With recent advances in the electron microscope, the MS lesions have been studied in detail. Research has discovered that these plaques are not uniform in composition and has placed them in four categories. Analysis of these categories suggests that there are two distinct pathways to myelin injury. In Patterns I and II, the myelin appears to be the target of an inflammatory mechanism, while in Patterns III and IV, oligodendrocytes (the cells that make the myelin sheaths for the nerve cells) are the target in what resembles a toxic, viral, or ischemic (lack of blood flow) process. In the case of axonal destruction, there is not much evidence, either accumulation of other cells or tissue, left at the scene of the crime.

Though plagued by symptoms, you may not be definitively diagnosed even though the words "multiple sclerosis" pop up with every visit and every professional. Do not let the lack of an official diagnosis, however, prevent you from starting the Recovery Diet—you have nothing to lose and everything to gain. The sooner in the disease you begin treatment, the easier it is to recover.

What's Happening?

Once you are diagnosed, what can you make of how this disease is working inside of you, beyond the manifestation of symptoms?

Bits and pieces of information about MS have been gathered and proven over time. They do not, however, fit into a complete, consistent picture. But these pieces can be useful and they are all that we have, in both the allopathic medical community and the alternative community. The following is the best theory about the disease mechanism of MS, given what is known about the disease.

Setting the Stage

Several precursors are set in place before MS manifests itself. Again, the picture is incomplete, but these appear to be the conditions:

VIRAL INFECTION AND T-CELL MEMORY

Extensive research suggests that there is a viral exposure before the age of fifteen to which the body reacts by setting the stage for attacking the self protein, myelin. Researchers are still looking for the viral culprit. But given that one definitive viral event has eluded scientists for decades, the process is probably not as simple as involving one virus or there being a direct link. Rather, like everything else about MS, it is more complicated and involved.

It is postulated that, as the result of this early infection, the immune system becomes improperly programmed, by which it does not differentiate self cells from external cells, attacking both. The T cells and the B cells are the immune system's fighters, specialized to attack foreign substances or antigens. Both of these cells are found in the plaques where myelin has been destroyed.

Taking it one step further, the proponents of the Recovery Diet suggest this confusion by the immune system is three-way. The virus, the myelin protein, and a sensitized food—usually rich in protein—are not differentiated by the immune cells; all are seen as external and thus attacked. This confusion of one minute substance for another is called molecular mimicry.

FAULTY BLOOD-BRAIN BARRIER (BBB)

Some malfunction occurs in the BBB, allowing the activated immune cells to cross into the CNS. In a normal person, the endothelial cells, the special cells lining the blood vessels along the nervous system, form an impenetrable shield to any foreign substance or cells that do not belong in the well-protected spinal fluid. In MS, this fail-safe protective system fails. The exact workings of the BBB, as well as the mechanism behind the failure to protect the nervous system, is not understood.

Dr. Roy Swank has extensively researched this aspect of MS; indeed, his dietary program is based on the theory that people with MS do not metabolize fats or lipids properly, allowing the formation of micro-embolisms. He proposes that the pressure these blood formations place on the smallest blood vessels next to the spinal cord causes the breach in the blood-brain barrier.

THE GENETIC CARD

Obviously, not everyone exposed to a virus as a child later develops MS. Studies have shown there to be some genetic predisposition, but it is far from being a major cause, only a contributing factor. People of northern European descent, especially Scandinavians, have a higher incidence of MS than other ethnic groups. Also, there is a higher incidence among family members and twins than in the general population, a fact that again gives credence to a genetic factor. There is a tie to the maternal line and families with MS also have a higher incidence of other autoimmune diseases.

ENVIRONMENT

The higher incidence of the disease in the northern climates suggests an environmental factor. This north-south gradient has been well documented over many decades.

But again, there are exceptions. Puzzling to researchers is the high incidence of MS in Sardinia, exceeding even that historically found in Scandinavia. The number of cases is increasing worldwide in adults, and tragically, young children are starting to manifest MS. Studies of MS in Japan and Thailand are showing disease profiles different from those in the West.

Another interesting phenomenon is the existence of clusters of a heightened incidence of MS in various locations. Studies have established that there is statistical significance to cluster areas found in Missouri, Illinois, Washington, and Texas. Science now has to discover why.

Smoking is one environmental factor definitively established as a risk.

Vitamin D as a protective factor has been established. This makes sense given that people in the southern climates, who are exposed to more sunlight (which provides Vitamin D), have a lower incidence of the disease than the people in the northern climates, who receive less sunlight.

DORMANCY

It is believed that a period of dormancy occurs between the initial event that lays down the template for MS and the actual first manifestation of symptoms. The length of this time span and even the reason there is dormancy are not understood. It is also possible that MS will never manifest, even though the precursors are all there.

More people are manifesting the disease, both earlier in childhood and later, beyond the historic fifty-year-old limit, raising questions about what has changed in our environment to cause this. Part of the answer might be in what we eat and the chemicals to which we are exposed.

There are cases in which extensive plaques or lesions are found in the brain or on the spinal cord during autopsy, yet no symptoms were ever manifested in the person's life. The discovery of the second disease process of axonal damage under normal-appearing white or gray matter helps to explain this phenomena. It also suggests, as many scientists suspect, that MS is more than one disease.

THE TRIGGER

Another unknown is what causes MS to manifest at a particular age or time in the person's life. The disease usually strikes between the ages of twenty and fifty, the most common being thirty or so, though the age range is widening considerably. There have been suggestions that trauma or stress triggers the disease, but nothing conclusive has resulted from the research.

Again as suggested above, the modern diet, common medications, and beverages have been shown to be damaging to the digestive system, especially in terms of maintaining the gut walls. If a degraded digestive system contributes to the manifestation of the disease, the modern diet might explain the recent appearance of MS at earlier ages.

Trouble Begins in the Central Nervous System

A person is vulnerable to having his or her MS triggered if there is genetic predisposition, an environmental exposure, a permeable blood-brain barrier, immune cells that have been sensitized to the self-protein of myelin, and an activation of immune cells.

On one level in an MS attack or exacerbation in Patterns I and II, the activated immune cells cross the blood-brain barrier into the CNS and identify the myelin as a foreign object. The body calls up a host of immune fighters that surround the site, which cause the inflammation ending in cell damage. At this site of destruction, the accumulated dead cells of the body and the immune system form hardened plaques, called sclerosis. Myelin may be stripped from around the nerves, and the nerve cells may be damaged or destroyed. The cells that are called in to repair and replace the myelin have been found in plaques as another casualty of this process. To add another layer of complication, it appears that some of the cells that cause the inflammation are the same ones that are protective in the aftermath—or the possibility exists that the inflammation is helpful in ending the disease episode, which again calls into question the treatment strategies that are designed to quell inflammation.

In Patterns III and IV, there appears to be another process, with the oligodendrocytes, the myelin makers, as targets and other cells streaming to the site to clean up. Upon examination of the plaques, complete descriptions of which cells are present are made, but it is not known which are causative and which appear as a result of the damage. Again, the T and other cells might serve a dual function.

On a second level, some research suggests that before any outward manifestation, axonal destruction begins under normal-appearing white or gray matter of the brain and spinal cord. This is the process which causes disability and appears to be continuous, despite the varying symptom profile or the inflammation load as reflected in the MRI lesions. There is little cellular matter found around the damaged axons, making the investigation of how and why this damage is occurring very difficult.

Over time, the disease may take many paths, leaving scars anywhere along the spinal cord or in the brain. Some sites of sclerosis will become dormant, while new lesions are born. There is no predictable course, but most often the disease progresses to some disability due to the second disease process of axonal damage. Researchers have noticed that after many years, when the person is quite old, the disease becomes quiescent, perhaps due to the normal weakening of the immune system. With so much damage already done by that time, it is of little comfort.

Research findings indicate that many other body chemicals or markers are modified in a person with MS: the cervical lymph nodes appear to play a role, saliva and blood show change, the amounts of some trace minerals are shown to be different in people with MS. Swank found that fat and lipid metabolism is compromised. Again, at this point all of these findings are only descriptive, but suggest that MS is a whole body disease or that the whole body works to fight it.

Are There Other Causes?

MS is basically an end point, a result of a disease process. There is a large amount of accumulated anecdotal evidence as well as some research that points to foods, but it is very possible that, in some individuals, other factors can activate the cascading events that end up as MS. Lyme disease resembles MS in its presentation—chronic inflammation and demyelination—but it has a known bacterial cause. Chronic rubella encephalitis, a rare reaction to the measles vaccination, also has the same disease process. New chemicals introduced into our environment, as well as heavy metals and viruses, may all possibly cause problems for an individual.

Demographics

Numerous studies all over the world show MS to be a disease of uneven distribution. Research of demographics, environmental factors, and genetics is again finding interesting facts, but no complete context as scientists troll for some clues to this disease.

Beyond genetics, there is a pattern in the distribution that correlates to that in diet. People living in those areas of highest incidence of MS rely heavily on dairy and grains. The central plains of Canada, where the wheat has the highest percentage of gluten, also have the highest incidence of MS. Studies have also traced migrations and the changing frequency of MS. Asians typically have a low incidence of MS, which increases when they move to Hawaii and then even more when they move to the mainland. Fishing villages in Norway have a lower incidence than the ones inland, where people rely more on dairy and wheat for their food. These studies do not decisively prove anything, but when combined with deductive reasoning are helpful in formulating an effective treatment approach.

For the Recovery Diet—Digestive System

The answer to how we become sensitized to certain foods lies in the digestive system's failure to maintain the integrity of its intestinal wall. "Leaky gut" is the term used for this condition, whose increasing incidence is shown by the number of people who find they can no longer eat one food or another.

In a healthy digestive system, there are colonies of microorganisms lining the digestive tract that aid in digestion and help protect the wall. Various substances we commonly ingest in modern life, like antibiotics, nonsteroidal anti-inflammatory drugs like aspirin and ibuprofen, alcohol, tobacco, and antacids kill these beneficial microorganisms. When you do need to take an antibiotic, it is important to restore these beneficial microorganisms with a probiotic.

A damaged gut allows small particles of partially digested food to pass into the bloodstream, instead of maintaining integrity and not allowing any food to pass until it is fully digested. The immune system quickly identifies and remembers these particles, which it sees as foreign invaders and then attacks. When that particular food is eaten subsequently, the immune system's memory will activate an immune cell attack again, thus creating food sensitivity. This is part of the reason food is key to recovering from MS.

All theories about MS agree that the immune cells are activated in the bloodstream before crossing the blood-brain barrier; the Recovery Diet recognizes that a major source of this activation is food.

What Can I Expect?

By the usual medical model, there is no one predictor of what course your MS will take. The range of outcomes is as individualized as everything else about this maddening disease. Science has set up four categories that describe the usual outcomes and their incidence.

1. ***Benign.*** This usually means there was one attack, often involving visual problems or numbness in one limb, with no permanent disability. Twenty percent of cases fit this category. This definition is not without some question. The American Academy of Neurology defines benign MS as someone having no symptoms with the subsequent discovery of lesions only upon autopsy. Given the discovery of a second layer of disease activity—the axonal loss—it may be that these cases are not MS at all. In other studies, using

the common definition of benign MS as first manifesting, then not showing any more progression, researchers have found unacknowledged loss in cognitive functions rather than the physical symptoms that mark the disease's continued destruction.

2. Relapse-remitting. In this type, a sudden onset of symptoms will be followed by a remission; this pattern repeats itself with no predictability over the years. Sometimes there is progressive disability, other times the person appears to be disease free. Twenty-four percent of the cases fit this description. The assumption that there is no disease activity in between exacerbations is called into question by the out-of-sight axonal damage. This type has been thought more amenable to some modification than the other types and is, therefore, the target of treatments. The goal of the treatments has been to reduce the inflammation in the CNS during manifestation of the transitory symptoms, which is difficult to validate given the quixotic and unpredictable nature of the disease. The outcome of these treatments has been measured by the reduction in lesion load and the decreased frequency of exacerbations, which have been shown to have no bearing on the ultimate outcome of disability. For unknown reasons, this type of MS usually evolves into secondary progressive at some time.

3. Relapse-progressive or secondary progressive. In this type, the effects from the attacks become cumulative, leaving some disability. And now it is known that the progressive degeneration occurs unabated through axonal damage under normal-appearing white and gray matter. There are no longer apparent full remissions. This is also the most common form of MS, with 40 percent of the cases fitting into this category.

4. Chronic progressive or primary progressive. From the first attack, the symptoms increase unabated to disability. Fortunately, this is the least common, at 15 percent. This is the least understood profile of MS.

There is no explanation for why a person has one type or another. The disease course is often initially relapsing-remitting, then turns secondary progressive at some point. No one understands why one person has one type and another person a more virulent or benign course.

You can be at any stage of this disease and still experience recovery and the elimination of symptoms following the MS Recovery Diet. The personal profiles of Part II illustrate how MS, in all degrees of progression, responds to this treatment with good results.

Conclusion

A safe conclusion is that MS is one or, possibly, many diseases in which there is destruction of the myelin sheath surrounding the nerves, causing a disruption of the electrical impulses. Along with this there is a second disease process of axonal destruction under both white and gray matter, which determines the disability. The exact nature or cause of either pathway is unknown. There is good research showing that the immune cells are activated by some antigen in the bloodstream before they cross the blood-brain barrier where the myelin is attacked. At least this comes close to explaining the inflammatory lesions of Patterns I and II. In Patterns III and IV, it is one of the immune system cells, the oligodendrocytes, that are the target of attack. This disruption caused by all or any of these disease pathways creates malfunctions, either in the form of minor symptoms or in major disabilities and everything in between.

MS is a whole-body disease, involving most bodily systems in either the disease process or in the body's attempt to fight the disease, even though it manifests in the nervous system. Following that same thinking, MS appears to be the result of a series of failures in many body systems, among them: a failure of the blood-brain barrier, the failure of the immune system to recognize self cells, a degenerative process of axonal destruction of unknown etiology, and an activation of the immune system on a regular basis. In the model used in the Recovery Diet, the failure of the digestive system leads to the creation of food sensitivities.

The human body is miraculous, and doesn't give in to MS without a fight. For example, there is evidence that when there is axonal or other nerve destruction, the cortex reorganizes, calling up other areas and cells to do the work of damaged areas. The body is a balance of tissue destruction, tissue repair, and cortical reorganization. The Recovery Diet works with the body, eliminating what causes harm and giving it the necessary tools to repair. It stops and reverses MS and restores full health.

2

The MS Recovery Diet

The first principle of the Recovery Diet is to stop ingesting the foods that activate the immune system and ultimately lead to symptoms. If the immune cells are not activated in the bloodstream they don't cross the blood-brain barrier into the CNS, and don't attack the myelin or activate axonal destruction, so no symptoms or disease mechanisms take place. Once you identify problem foods and eliminate them from the diet, disease activity stops or greatly diminishes.

The second principle is to consciously ingest those foods that have been shown to aid in healing. When the disease stops, the body will heal from even the most progressed cases of MS.

In summary, there are foods that harm and others that heal. You need to modify your diet to eliminate the first and add sufficient amounts of the second for a complete recovery.

Of the many factors that play a role in the manifestation of MS—genetics, environment, an early viral incident, the false programming of the immune system, blood-brain barrier failure of unknown etiology—only food is under our control. Without having to solve all the mysteries of the body, specifically the nervous, immune, and vascular systems, the simple act of changing your diet can accomplish all that is needed to recover.

We now understand that MS is a multisystem problem, and for each person affected, the disease manifests in a unique constellation of symptoms, pattern of progression, and degree of severity. It follows logically then that an effective treatment must also be multifaceted and specific to the individual. You will need to listen to your body and tailor the general program to meet your particular disease profile. As MS is a disease of daily changes, it follows that a contributing factor also reflects daily changes. In the case of MS it is food. The diet is not a cure, but that is irrelevant when a complete cessation of symptoms and a return to health are the results.

Which Foods?

There are five food groups that are most often implicated to one degree or another in the disease process for most people. Along with those general foods, other specific foods of any type to which you have become sensitized through leaky gut or some other mechanism are also triggers. All of these offending foods need to be identified and eliminated from your diet.

The existing theory that explains why these food groups—dairy, gluten grains, legumes, eggs, and yeast—are most problematic goes back in mankind's history over the two million years of human development. During most of this time, humans have adapted and evolved on the Paleolithic diet, namely wild meats, fish, nuts, vegetables, and fruits. Relatively recently in human history, about 12,000 years ago, dairy and grains were added as agriculture and animal husbandry began, first in the Middle East and then spreading northward and westward, reaching Scandinavia and the British Isles about 6,000 years ago. One theory suggests that, with less time to adapt to these relatively new foods, the people of northern Europe developed a much higher incidence of MS than the people in the Middle East. Beyond MS, the Paleolithic diet is more healthful, and following it reduces the risk for other diseases of modern man, such as heart disease, diabetes, and some cancers.

For those with MS, all five of these protein-rich foods should be held suspect as potential culprits. Not all people with MS are sensitive to all five—dairy, grains containing gluten, legumes, eggs, and yeast. Some find they are highly sensitive to dairy, others to gluten grains, and others to a combination. For example, Roger MacDougall was highly sensitive to grains and made a remarkable recovery eliminating them as well as sugar and fats. It soon became evident to the people who followed his diet that other foods beyond gluten-containing grains, fats, and sugars were triggers for MS symptoms, and MacDougall integrated that discovery into his later writings.

To avoid problems, it is helpful to understand more about the five groups:

Dairy is often a problem to MS patients. Beyond that, a significant percentage of the world's population is lactose intolerant.

Grains containing gluten include wheat, rye, and barley. Oats are sometimes considered to contain gluten and sometimes not, so each person should check his or her own tolerance. All grains can potentially be troublesome, even rice, though it appears to be the safest. Read labels carefully, checking for modified food starch, which is often wheat based.

Legumes are the family of plants that returns nitrogen to the soil. They include beans like limas and red beans, for example, as well as peanuts and soybeans. Tofu is a soy product, so be cautious.

Eggs are often used in unexpected places, e.g., as a thickener in salad dressing.

Yeast is the easiest to identify and seems to be the least common offender.

But beyond the five usual suspects, each person may have very individual food sensitivities to herbs, spices, or food in any category. These can be obvious in their immediate reaction with resulting symptoms, or more elusive in delayed reactions. Food sensitivities or allergies are the reaction of the immune system to antigens, foreign bodies which in this case are foods. There are five major types of immunoglobulin, an antibody produced in response to a perceived antigen: IgE, IgG, IgA, IgM, and IgD. The IgE is the antibody identified in the classic allergic reaction and is the focus of the common skin scratch test. Its reaction is immediate and measurable. IgG's involvement, while slower to show, also is implicated in producing symptoms.

In both the general food categories and the individual sensitivities, it is the immune response that identifies specific foods that trigger your symptoms.

Saturated fat and sugar are also foods that should be avoided. Because of the poor metabolizing of fat by people with MS, the ingestion of saturated fat contributes to the breaches in the blood-brain barrier. And sugar's corrosive nature compromises the body's barriers as well. This is explained further in the section below.

Pinpointing Your Food Sensitivities

Over time, as your symptoms diminish and become discrete, finite events, your offending foods become very apparent. At the beginning, a certain amount of guesswork and experimentation is necessary in getting to know exactly which foods are your triggers. To start, various methods can be used to test for food sensitivities. The three most reliable, which are scientifically based, are skin testing, the RAST or ELISA tests, and individual food challenges.

In a skin test you can see the IgE antibody reaction of the immune system, specifically an instantaneous inflammation of the skin. The medical technician will scratch your skin with various food molecules and watch for reddened swelling to appear. This is a classic allergy test, which also measures response to pollens, animal dander, and other chemicals. The drawback is that the reaction of one antibody, the IgE, is measured, ignoring the slower or more subtle reactions of the other immunoglobulins, which can also be activated. All of these activated immune cells can cross the blood-brain barrier and cause MS symptoms.

The second method for identifying the immune-reactive foods

involves introducing the food in question to a blood sample and observing and counting the immune cell activation. Both the RAST (Radio-allergosorbent) and the ELISA (enzyme-linked immunosorbent assay) tests do this. These tests measure both the IgE and the IgG antibody reactions. Though these tests are prone to error with false negatives and false positives occurring, they do give you a rough guideline with which to start.

The weakness in these two tests is that the strength of the reaction by the immune cells to a particular food is partially dependent on how recently and how much of this food has been eaten. For example, if you haven't ingested wheat for months, your immune system's memory of it as an antigen would fade and might not react with just one introduction to it. Whereas another food might be just a mild problem, but if you ate a lot before the test, the immune system memory would be fresh and react with more vigor than might actually be the case overall.

The third method is for the MS patient to methodically test each food, which is done by starting with a diet of a limited number of known safe, nonreactive foods, then adding back one food at a time and observing the reaction. This method is tedious and time consuming, but you get to know your body and all its reactions.

Again, over time it becomes easier to identify the offending foods. If after a meal you experience a reaction such as numb tingling, a fleeting spasm, or some other telltale sign, you can make an account of the foods you ingested. Then at a later time, these foods can be tested for reactions, by eating them with all known safe foods and seeing if there is a reaction. It is in developing a greater sensitivity to their bodies that people with MS can understand and fine-tune their individual food programs.

As previously mentioned, food allergies/sensitivities are more complex than the instantaneous reaction of the IgE antibodies. Sometimes, it takes hours or even a day for people to react to a troublesome food, which makes it harder for them to identify the culprit or even recognize that their problem might be an allergy. As a result, many people suffer from a food allergy/sensitivity and don't know it. And not all food sensitivities can be explained. It may be that there are nonallergenic mediated food sensitivities, reflecting our individual tolerance for certain foods. These cannot be measured by any test, but must be ferreted out by the individuals through careful observation of their reactions to specific foods.

Complicating this is the little understood phenomenon referred to as an addictive allergy, whereby the individual craves the very food to which he or she has a negative reaction. The root cause of craving foods that are destructive to you may lie in the body's inability to completely digest those foods. Yet for normal functioning and maintenance, the body requires a certain level of nutrients and will send out a signal to the mind to get these nutrients even if they are in harmful foods. So, the body is in the trap of craving foods that it is allergic to, leading to more symptoms. This is an addictive allergy, so be careful and watch when you crave certain foods.

Illness activates the immune system, which then can trigger symptoms. Likewise, stress and fatigue can result in a flare-up of symptoms. Over time, as you recover and get stronger, these conditions will no longer affect the disease.

You will find that identifying your trigger foods will naturally evolve as you follow the diet. You don't need to stop ingesting all of them to see improvement, and as you improve and get to know your body, it will become clear to you which foods are causing symptoms. When you are close to full recovery, it will be a matter of fine-tuning and eliminating those foods that cause just subtle reactions.

Other Culprits—Fat And Sugar

Fat and sugar, America's favorite ingredients, also contribute to the manifestation of MS.

Again, reflecting the principles of Paleolithic nutrition, saturated fat is implicated in the erosion of the blood-brain barrier. Dr. Roy Swank researched the role saturated fat plays in MS at the microcirculatory level. He postulated that people with MS do not process saturated fats efficiently and that embolisms of these fats form in the bloodstream and put pressure on the microcirculatory system, which eventually leads to a breach in the blood-brain barrier. From the early 1950s to well into the 1990s, Dr. Swank followed patients who used his low-fat, high-oil diet prescription. From his work it is now well known that severely limiting the intake of saturated fats is beneficial in halting or slowing the progression of MS. His guideline stipulates that a maximum of 15 grams, or 1 teaspoon, of saturated fat should be consumed each day. To meet this guideline, red meat needs to be just about eliminated from the diet. Dr. Swank allows for one small serving a week. This is stringent, since even a tablespoon of the healthiest oil usually contains at least 1 gram of saturated fat. It is important that even these hidden sources, like the 2 grams in a serving of olive oil or the several grams in a handful of almonds, be counted.

As Dr. Swank's research progressed, he discovered the importance of the essential fatty acids, which are the healthy oils. Dr. Swank recommends that four to ten teaspoons of unsaturated and monounsaturated oil be ingested daily. These are the omega-3-rich oils like fish and flaxseed oil; sunflower, safflower, grape seed, and walnut oils, which are high in omega-6; and olive oil, high in the omega-9s.

For a person whose MS has just recently appeared, limiting fat and adding healthy oils (essential fatty acids) may be sufficient to halt and reverse MS.

Sugar also contributes to symptoms, as identified early on by MacDougall. Again, sugar was not part of the Paleolithic diet and has been shown to be corrosive to the capillary walls, well noted in people with diabetes. Sugar also often shows up on the tests as a food allergy. It is something to be suspected as contributing to symptoms and should be carefully observed to determine the MS person's tolerance for it. Note that sugar comes in many forms—sucrose, glucose, and fructose—all of which need to be monitored for reactions. High-fructose corn syrup is a major ingredient in the modern American diet.

Cravings for sugar and starches are common and understandable once we learn how the body balances sugars. For those with MS, it is crucial to maintain the right sugar balance in the body because too much sugar can cause symptoms. If your usual fare is sugary or starchy food, then you experience a sugar spike followed by an equally sharp fall in glucose levels. This drop will cause you to crave more sugar and the cycle will continue—not just affecting your MS, but your mood, and putting you at risk for other health problems, such as diabetes.

Note that fruits might have to be limited due to reactions to fructose, and there may be other restrictions unique to each individual. Follow the wisdom of your body.

Sometimes there is confusion when we speak of protein foods as common triggers, which is true for the grains, dairy, eggs, and legumes. However, lean protein such as poultry, fish, and wild game has not been found to be a source of problems for people with MS. Even beef is not usually an antigen; the prohibition against red meat is due only to its high fat content.

Starting the Recovery Diet

Eliminating the Foods That Harm

The first step is to avoid all the foods that trigger symptoms. You may want to be tested for food sensitivities first to give you a rough idea of the foods to which you are uniquely sensitive. Keep in mind, however, that these tests may give you an incomplete picture.

Stopping all potentially offending foods at once is difficult and hard on the body. Our bodies get used to a certain way of eating, and a drastic change can result in digestive and elimination problems. Plus, avoiding all foods at once doesn't give you as much information as you get with gradual eliminations. The exception to this suggestion would be if your MS is so advanced and your symptoms so severe that you can't differentiate small changes in day-to-day symptoms. In this case, it is probably best to at least eliminate all of the usual suspects from your diet. When your symptoms have sufficiently abated so you can differentiate reactions, then you might want to test each of the five main culprits. The other potential problem with the gradual approach is for people whose body needs to do some healing before any diminishing of symptoms appears. If over the weeks of gradually eliminating one food group and another you find there is no difference, you might be advised to eliminate them all with the assumption that other healing will take place first. Don't lose faith in the efficacy of this diet. Some people have strictly followed the diet for over a year before getting results, but it is worth it in the recovery they obtained for the rest of their lives.

Start by eliminating wheat and gluten for a week or two and see if you get any results. Next cut out dairy, the other most common problem food, followed by eggs, legumes, and yeast. When symptoms diminish, keep avoiding that food at all times. With regard to the other food groups, continue to watch and monitor.

Keeping a food diary helps in tracking food in relation to symptoms. You will record as well as see and feel patterns. If your symptoms usually flare in the afternoon, study your lunches, whereas if your symptoms appear at night or in the morning, check and evaluate what you are eating for dinner. As your symptoms diminish, it becomes easier to know exactly what is triggering your responses.

Along with eliminating suspected foods, keep your saturated fat to 15 grams a day and keep sugar ingestion to a minimum.

Ways to Improve Digestion

After you make the dietary changes necessary to eliminate the food allergens, the next strategy is to work on improving digestion. Foods become allergens when the gut is impaired. Infections, candida overgrowth, trauma, alcohol consumption, the use of certain medications, especially NSAIDs, smoking, poor nutrition, as well as continued ingestion of allergenic foods are all causal factors. You may want to explore this possibility with a health professional. A strong, intact intestinal lining will stop food particles from entering the bloodstream, preventing foods from becoming allergens and also keeping other harmful substances out. Also, it is important that food move through the digestive tract optimally to minimize the toxins that are absorbed.

In order to reestablish intestinal health, it is important first to stop doing things that are damaging. Thus you'll need to:

1. Cut down on the use of the group of medicines classified as nonsteroid anti-inflammatory drugs, like aspirin and ibuprofen (NSAIDs).
2. Cut back on the use of alcohol, and stop smoking.
3. Cut back on the use of antacids. It is our stomach acids that fight intestinal infections, which can harm intestinal walls.
4. Use antibiotics wisely. Antibiotics are correctly named; they kill the microorganisms in our bodies. Unfortunately, they do not distinguish between the harmful and beneficial microbes, like the flora in our gut that is helpful to us. When these are destroyed, the harmful bacteria that we ingest daily with our food have room to establish themselves in our intestines. If you do take antibiotics, be sure to replenish your digestive tract with the beneficial microbes, like lactobacillus acidophilus and lactobacillus bulgaricus. These are sold as supplements under those names or as combination probiotics.

It is important to do these positive actions that support the integrity of the digestive tract:

1. Chew your food thoroughly. By chewing, you not only give the digestive process a good start by utilizing the incredible strength of the teeth to grind the food up into more manageable bits, but you also generate saliva, which contains enzymes that start the digestive process. Another helpful factor is the enzyme in the saliva called the epidermal growth factor, which is both protective and healing to the gut.
2. Eat a high-fiber, healthy diet consisting mainly of fruits, vegetables, low-fat proteins, and nuts. This is basically the Paleolithic

diet to which our bodies are best suited. This dietary regime not only will supply the needed nutrients for healthy maintenance, but will also provide adequate fiber to keep the foods moving through the digestive tract.

3. Use oils, not fats. The essential fatty acids, like fish oil and flaxseed, safflower, sunflower, olive, and canola oils, which contain omega-3 and omega-6, help maintain the intestinal lining. Flaxseed and deep-sea cold-water fish are especially high in omega-3. Olive oil is primarily omega-9, which is also healthy.

4. Keep a healthy level of good microbes in your system.

Once the Disease Process Is Stopped, Repair Begins

Symptoms will fade and disappear and full functioning will be restored in MS. Remember, this is only possible after a great deal of repair and restoration within our bodies. We know which systems have failed—the blood-brain barrier, the immune system, and the nervous system, specifically in the destruction of myelin and nerve fibers—so it is safe to assume that part of the recovery reflects healing in these systems.

Though much remains a mystery, we know enough about these systems to be able to identify what foods and nutrients can aid in their repair. It follows logically that we should include these healing foods in our diets.

BLOOD-BRAIN BARRIER

In general, it is thought that free radicals damage the blood-brain barrier. Studies show that three related chemicals—anthocyanosides, proanthocyanidins, and oligomers—make this barrier more impermeable. They not only bind with the barrier, but are also powerful antioxidants. These chemicals are found in most foods, especially in brightly colored fruits and vegetables, wine, and tea. The berries and grapes are especially good sources (see Appendix A). The essential fatty acids also serve to strengthen the blood-brain barrier, as well as the digestive tract.

IMMUNE SYSTEM

At least partly, MS is classified as an autoimmune disease, which is the result of an overactive, overresponsive immune system. Specifically, the suppression side of the immune system, which is programmed to shut down the harmful autoimmune attacks against the self, needs to be restored. Several mechanisms and necessary ingredients to dampen the immune reactions have been identified—especially, the roles of fats and oils and of vitamin D.

1. *Fats and Oils.* A group of chemicals made by the body called prostaglandins (PG) serve to help regulate the immune system. Of the three main groups of PGs, PG1 and PG3 are immune suppressors, while PG2 signals the immune system to become more active. The body cannot manufacture these chemicals without ingesting the raw ingredients. All the PGs are derived from dietary fat, but interestingly, the suppressor PGs are made from the essential fatty acids. These are found in certain oils—fish, vegetable, nut, and seed. The immune-activating PGs are derived from animal fat found in red meat and dairy.

   Again, especially in the case of MS, it is important to limit saturated fat in the diet and, at the same time, to ingest a healthy amount of the oils to calm the overactive immune system.

2. *Vitamin D.* This vitamin provides several immune regulatory functions, among them suppressing antibody production and limiting inflammatory reactions. In short, it dampens the autoimmune response and keeps inflammation down.

The best source of vitamin D is sunlight. It is probably no coincidence that MS is more prevalent in the northern climates where there is less sun, especially in the winter months. Studies have shown there is a higher mortality for people with MS who have less sun exposure. Of course, science has also shown sun exposure to be cancer causing, so prudence is the key. This vitamin is also found in fish oil.

MYELIN AND NERVES

The body does repair and replace myelin, but in most MS cases, the rate of inflammation and destruction exceeds the body's capacity to repair and replace. The diet/nutritional treatment, over time, slows or halts the disease process, allowing the body to make progress in the repair and replacement of the myelin, and also to stop the axon destruction and allow for repair there as well. But it is important to insure that the body has the essential ingredients to repair and replace the myelin to the fullest extent possible. Two nutrients are crucial to myelin repair:

Vitamin B_{12} has many functions within the body, one of the most important being the formation and maintenance of myelin.

Lecithin is a major fat found in the cell membranes, in part because of the chemical phosphatidylserine.

Nongluten grains and liver are good sources for vitamin B_{12}, while lecithin is made in the body from a healthy balanced diet.

So When Am I Going to Start Feeling Better?

There is a great variation after starting the Recovery Diet and when you'll see results. It took Roger MacDougall some time before he saw any improvement. He wrote: "The results were very slow in coming; logic told me that the myelin sheath was probably a more complex tissue to repair than, say, simple flesh." Symptoms often appear as the last stage of any disease's progression, so too, much healing might need to take place before symptoms finally disappear: the last to arrive and the last to leave. Patience is the key. Nothing will happen overnight and improvement often comes in almost imperceptible steps.

Recovery Progresses

After a certain amount of time that varies with each person, the disease stops progressing. Though it is not understood how, the second disease path of axonal destruction, under the normal-appearing white and gray matter, also stops, as evidenced by the complete cessation of symptoms and return to full functioning of the people who have followed this treatment program.

With the progression stopped and some recovery started, you will probably lose your fear of the disease and feel more confident in what you are doing. Also, by this time you will know your body and be able to read its subtle signs. Being your own science lab serves a good purpose—you become the expert on your own disease and how it acts on your body. Armed with all this knowledge and skills, you can begin to experiment more with your diet.

After recovery is established, the fact that the immune cells will forget an antigen allows for the return of certain foods to your diet, especially if they are eaten in moderation and rotation. Rotating foods keeps the immune system's memory from placing that food high on the threat list, therefore not activating in response to the appearance of that food at four- or five-day intervals. There are some foods that you many never again eat, but that is not always the case. As with all facets of MS, this is highly idiopathic. Some people have returned to eating everything with impunity, while others continue to have prohibitions. Being careful not to damage the digestive system again is important for the return to more normal, though still very healthy, eating.

At this stage of recovery, if a symptom does flare, drinking a lot of water and exercising helps to work it through and out of the body faster.

As the saying goes, the best defense is a good offense. In the case of MS, the best strategy is having a healthy, rested, fit, and unstressed body. Rarely do exacerbations appear out of nowhere; stress and trauma are often the precipitators.

Exercise is important to keep muscles toned, stress low, and all systems functioning at their best. Dr. Swank recommends exercise to keep the blood moving, relieving pressure on the microcirculatory system. This in turn will keep the blood from pooling in the venules and causing breaches in the blood-brain barrier. Yoga has been shown to be beneficial in developing better balance, maintaining flexibility, increasing muscle tone as well as for general relaxation.

Rest is important to fight multisystem failure as well as plain fatigue associated with MS, but it also helps to keep the daily fluctuations of symptoms to a minimum.

The Importance of Attitude

Everyone we talked to who has healed spoke of the importance of attitude. In response to their disease, each of these people decided that they were not going to be, or stay, disabled. Their belief in their own power, and the power of their bodies to heal, was greater than any fear they had of the disease. Trust in a greater power and a deep spirituality was also common in the people we talked to as an important factor in their healing. Along the same line, all those who had healed felt they had become better people by having the disease. Rather than bitterness, they all expressed gratitude for the experience.

Through very effective fund-raising campaigns, an image of MS has been burned into the consciousness of most Americans: a young adult tragically confined to a wheelchair, smiling bravely. Also, the universal perception is that MS will inevitably progress to more disability. This pervasive image of MS works on the minds of people diagnosed with the disease. If attitude is crucial, then the pessimism and fatalism of prevailing thought works against an attitude of healing. Instead, there is the risk of it becoming a self-fulfilling prophecy as the person becomes identified with the disease.

A neurologist was overheard saying that it didn't matter what you did, since with MS you were only going to get worse. To his mind, anyone with MS was going to go downhill in their functioning. If you accept and integrate his attitude, you would not have had the energy or the faith to pursue an independent healing path.

Healing is very empowering and confidence boosting, while disability robs people of a sense of value, worth, and power. As small improvements in the course of the disease spur individuals on the healing path to redouble their efforts, an increase in symptoms pushes the already emotionally depleted person with MS to stop trying, risking greater disability and furthering their decline.

In the end, each person with MS forms his or her own unique relationship with the disease. No matter how progressed the disease, we all have the freedom of choice in attitude. In the battle against MS, choosing a positive attitude can make a big difference.

A Note on Supplements

There are many supplements that potentially can help in the battle against MS, but there is no universal opinion on their use. Dr. Swank feels that only a good multiple vitamin is necessary, while the ARMS group in England, through which the diet approach also evolved, feels that no supplements are needed. To get enough of the B vitamins, they recommend eating up to a pound of liver a week. Though this may be good from the vitamin B standpoint, there are concerns about the amount of toxins in animal livers due to modern farming methods and the chemicals that are introduced. Again, how you want to approach the issue of supplements is a matter for experimentation to determine which are helpful to the specific individual. The supplements usually recommended fall into several categories: The essential fatty acids and oils, vitamins, minerals, antioxidants, enzymes, probiotics, and amino acids. A list of possibly helpful supplements can be found in Appendix A.

Summary

The Recovery Diet treatment addresses all the components of the MS disease process. This approach illustrates how much our bodies have evolved to use a certain nutritional regime, namely the Paleolithic diet. Most of the many contributing factors we have no control over; it happened in the past, is part of our DNA, or is unknown. What is certain is that the immune system is activated before it crosses the blood-brain barrier and wreaks havoc in the CNS. Given that food is one of the main things that can activate the immune system, it is one area where we can stop the sequence of events that leads to the inflammation and destruction of the myelin or the axonal damage that characterizes MS. We can control what we eat.

To take the path to healing, it is important that people with MS adhere strictly to the specific nutritional regime that works for them.

1. Suspect and investigate dairy, gluten-containing grains, legumes, eggs, and yeast as possible allergens and eliminate them from your diet.
2. Avoid all other allergenic foods that you have identified as triggers.
3. Limit saturated fats, processed sugar, alcohol, and caffeine. Stop smoking.
4. Eat fish, skinless breast of chicken or turkey, wild game or other low-fat animal meat, and nuts for protein, fruits and vegetables for carbohydrates and micronutrients. Also use oils such as flaxseed, olive, and sunflower, which are polyunsaturated and monounsaturated.
5. Limit use of NSAIDs and antacids. Use antibiotics judiciously. After use, replace gut microbes with probiotics.
6. Chew your food thoroughly. Eat plenty of fruits and vegetables.
7. Eat a lot of flavonoid-rich foods like blueberries and cherries.

8. Spend some time in the sun.
9. Get plenty of rest.
10. Exercise.
11. Reduce stress.

Taking the Plunge

The beauty of the Recovery Diet is that it works, despite all the questions that remain about this puzzling disease. This diet/nutritional program alone has shown to give true healing and recovery. We hope that science will solve the puzzle of MS, but that looks to be many years away. In the meantime, the diet offers reversal, healing, and recovery from the ravages of this disease.

The potential rewards of following this healing path are great, the risks are none, but it is a challenge. The diet demands strict adherence, patience, and discipline. The modern way of life and eating are in antithesis to its main tenets, but that road is proving with each passing year to be the road to disease and poor health.

Taking the plunge will bring you into a new world of eating and way of relating to your body. You'll make wonderful discoveries about yourself and the hold MS has on your life will diminish. Welcome to this new world, and good luck!

3

MS: A Short, Perplexing History

Throughout the entire history of multiple sclerosis, the disease has baffled researchers and thwarted all attempts to unlock its secrets. From when it was first identified some one hundred fifty years ago, speculation about the nature of the disease has variously defined MS as a vascular disease, an infectious disease, a genetic disease, an environmental disease, an allergic disease, an inflammatory disease, and an autoimmune disease. It is probably all of these and more.

A Late Beginning

A modern disease, MS evidently did not appear until the nineteenth century. Among its early victims, some experts believe, were the German poet Heinrich Heine and Augustus d'Este, an illegitimate grandson of George III of England. After a similar twenty-five-year course, both men died in the mid-1800s.

When medical science progressed through the use of autopsies, "disseminated sclerosis" was first identified as a unique disease entity. Previously it had been associated with syphilis. Jean Cruveilhier, in his book *Anatomie Pathologique du Corps Humain* (1829–1842), illustrated the hallmark scarring of MS along the CNS. Jean-Martin Charcot, another French medical pioneer, first named the diagnostic triad of nystagmus (spasmodic motion of the eyeball), intention tremors (tremors that appear only when there is movement, rather than all the time), and scanning speech for what is now known as MS.

As increasing numbers of cases were identified, the description of the disease became more complete and uniform. In 1856, the German physician Friedrich Theodor von Frerichs listed the following: the condition is produced gradually with exacerbations and remissions, one side of the body is first affected, paresis of the lower extremities appears early and reaches a high degree, and the disturbances of motility outweigh those of sensibility.

Treatment was left to the individual physician, who would prescribe his own concoctions with ingredients such as quicksilver (mercury), arsenic, and iodine.

New understanding and insight were added piecemeal, but there were no major breakthroughs by 1920. Demographic patterns were observed, such as the rate of incidence of MS was greater in Scandinavia, in women, and in young adults. The possible link to an early childhood infection was made and the search for that one infectious agent, be it bacterial or viral, was begun and continues to this day.

Theory focused on the swelling or inflammation of the myelin substance, after which the myelin was thought to be permanently altered. Vascular changes, such as the presence of venules, or microscopic blood vessels, at the scarring sites, were observed. "It is not improbable that vasospasm is a manifestation of toxic or allergic process," Drs. Woltman, Merritt, and Houston wrote in a 1948 publication of the Association for Research in Nervous and Mental Disorders.

Since the late 1940s and early 1950s, fat and faulty lipid metabolism, which clog and pressure the microvessels in the vascular system, were identified as causative factors. Dr. Roy Swank and others continued to research and write about dietary treatments for MS, with their findings presented in medical journals. In a 1973 issue of the *British Medical Journal*, J. H. D. Miller and colleagues reported the positive results of research on the efficacy of sunflower seed oil. They "established an important landmark in the history of MS in reporting that supplementation of the diet with sunflower seed oil, in a properly controlled, double-blind trial over the space of two years, had a statistically significant effect in reducing the number and severity of MS exacerbations (though not the gradual downward trend)."

Dr. Swank, who ran an MS clinic in Portland, Oregon, after bringing his study of the disease from Canada, continued work on the role of fats, saturated as well as the oils, in multiple sclerosis. Mainstream medicine diverged to other theories and treatments.

Swank guided patients in a dietary treatment approach based mostly on the theory that faulty fat metabolism in people with MS created microscopic emboli (clots of blood), which exerted pressure on the capillaries causing the blood-brain barrier to be breached. He followed patients on a low-fat diet for more than forty years, all the while keeping data on their improvements. Over time, he refined this treatment to include an increased ingestion of the essential fatty acids (4–10 teaspoons a day) versus a limit of less than 15 grams of saturated fat a day. His findings showed better results in retarding MS than any other treatment had shown to date. Though he was an M.D. and had scientific articles published on a regular basis in all the respected medical journals, Swank's conclusions were never integrated into mainstream medical theory or practice. One rationale given for not embracing his conclusions was that he did not have a control group. Swank's response was that it would be unethical to have a control group, denying them the benefits of a treatment he knew to work.

Dr. Swank had a remarkable career, spanning from the early 1950s, when he began studying the role of fat in MS, to his retirement more than four decades later. His *Muliple Sclerosis Diet Book*, cowritten with Barbara Brewer Dugan, is still a top seller among books about the disease.

Allergy was also named as a contributing factor. Ingestion of certain foods was connected to the allergic response in the post–World War II years. Dr. Richard Brichener stated that there was a "distinct influence on the cause of the disease exercised by the administration of grain," in a 1948 publication of the Association for Research in Nervous and Mental Disorders, which reviewed all the latest research of that year. The connection of MS to food sensitivities was widely accepted at this time. Treatments recommended by Dr. Putnam of Harvard included: avoiding foods that were not tolerated, using anticoagulants, improving nutrition, rehabilitating symptoms, and psychotherapy.

Roger MacDougall, a screenwriter and award-winning playwright, was first diagnosed with MS in 1953. By the 1970s, he had deteriorated to the point of being unable to stand, having also lost his vision, as well as the use of his hands and legs. He refused to accept that his condition was hopeless. Lying in bed, he began thinking about his disease and decided to take responsibility for his health into his own hands.

Using logic, he drew upon the knowledge of other degenerative diseases and their tie-in to foods. Looking at celiac disease (a digestive disease) and gluten, diabetes and sugar, heart disease and animal fat, he noticed that these disease-causing foods were historically more recent additions to the human diet. He eliminated these foods from his diet and ate a more natural, whole-food diet. Though his symptoms stabilized, it took years before he experienced significant improvement. He persisted, refining his understanding, noting that he also needed to make up the deficits of nutrients in his body, adding in the foods that heal as well as eliminating the foods that harm. When he died, well into his eighties, he was symptom-free.

MacDougall generously shared his experience in his writings. Many others followed his diet, experiencing the same success. At first, MacDougall had identified only wheat, sugar, and fat as the culprits, avoidance of which fortunately led to his recovery. Many people who followed his program had the same success, but there were also many who didn't improve. MacDougall then realized that each person was unique and that not all people were allergic or sensitive to the same foods as he was.

He summed up his understanding of MS this way: "Is it not possible that there are no causes other than the autonomous breakdown in each victim of cell tissue—a process which presupposes no disease-causing mechanism but can be explained quite handily as the result of metabolic imbalance, the effect of an allergic reaction to some foods, or to some vitamin and mineral deficiency?"

He continued to write and spread the word about this treatment, even selling a vitamin combination that he developed, helping many people recover. But since his message had not been integrated into the institutions of medicine and health, his message did not grow and spread after his death. Nor did any of the institutions of medicine or research follow up with studies of his treatment program.

Many people have healed using the concepts of MacDougall and Swank. And these people, who succeeded in healing, often sought to share the good news in any way they could. One such effort is a pamphlet written by J. C. Ogilvie, who describes his progress of recovering from long-term, disabling MS. Another is John Pageler, who began his recovery by visiting Dr. Swank, and subsequently sent out countless newsletters to MS sufferers advocating the diet approach. Almost universally, when people find a method for recovery, they try to share it. Without the formal organization and structures of the medical establishment, disseminating this knowledge has been hit or miss. In recent years, the advent of the Internet has made information sharing easier and more efficient.

Ashton Embry, at the website Direct-MS.org, has assembled much of the latest information and research that supports the dietary approach. He has also worked at raising money to fund much-needed research into the dietary approach.

Divergence

Beginning in the 1960s and 1970s, allopathic medicine diverged from allergy and fat metabolism as contributing causes of MS. There were no definitive studies to discredit these ideas, but neither of these approaches was yielding the type of cure that was expected of medicine.

With better understanding of the inflammatory process and improved technology, allopathic medicine turned its attentions to other aspects of the immune system and the development of medicines to alter its actions. The first immune-modifying agents discovered were the steroids. Since steroids can be used to suppress the immune system, they became the treatment of choice. This treatment has proven effective in muting and ending exacerbations and is used to this day. However, it was found that long-term usage had more risks than rewards; these drugs are now used for acute treatment only.

Cancer treatments, the chemotherapy cocktails, also act on the immune system and have shown to have some benefit to people with MS, again more as a short-term intervention. These, too, are problematic, with risks to the heart and can only be used sparingly.

Scientists kept searching for something that would prove truly effective for the long term. The next discovery was that the interferons, produced in the body, regulate the immune system—some activating it; others dampening it. Specifically, interferons have been found to decrease inflammation and swelling, as well as slow the proliferations of T cells and B cells in the immune system. Researchers were able to engineer interferons, mainly the beta interferon, specifically for MS. Betaseron, Avonex, and Rebif are interferon drugs put on the market in the 1990s. These were soon followed by the introduction of another drug, Copaxone, a substance similar to myelin, based on the theory that immune cells would attack these decoy cells instead of the real myelin.

These drugs were declared the major breakthrough everyone had been waiting for, and all hope rested on these medications to finally offer some relief to people with MS.

Sadly, these drugs have not lived up to the original hope, though their ineffectiveness has not been as widely publicized as the original promises were years before. Consistent with all aspects of MS, no one drug proved to be effective with all people; some people responded well, while others did not respond at all or had many side effects. Unanticipated in the research, a high percentage of people developed antibodies to the drugs themselves, negating any effectiveness. A 2006 article in *Current Medical Opinion and Research* states: "The induction of NAbs (Neutralizing Antibodies) in IFN-beta (Avonex, Betaseron, Rebif) treated patients reduces clinical effect and accelerates disease progression." The same problems have been encountered with Copaxone, though it is a different drug type entirely.

In an issue of *Current Opinion in Neurology* in 2006, a group of doctors from the Mayo Clinic wrote: "It is difficult to prove long-term benefit of therapy in chronic disease characterized by individual variability and unpredictability and there exists no study that convincingly establishes a long-term improvement over natural history for any MS therapy."

A new drug was next developed whose action is to prevent the activated immune cells from passing through the blood-brain barrier: Natalizumab, a monoclonal antibody, marketed as Tysabri. The drug binds the immune cells, which prevents the cells from crossing the blood-brain barrier into the CNS. Though most effective of all drugs developed so far, there are also risks of death and infection. Tysabri was taken off the market after two patients died. After researchers studied the risk/reward balance, it was decided to put the drug back on the market.

Steroids and the cancer drugs also continue to be used. Genetic modification and stem cell therapy are being intensely researched as possible answers. Other drugs being considered now are: an Alzheimer's drug, Donepezil; statins for vascular protection; and intravenous immunoglobin.

Much of the new research adds more questions and confusion about MS than points toward a cure. Now it is known that there are four types of plaques with apparently two distinct disease mechanisms, and there is a second disease path of axonal destruction of unknown etiology under normal-appearing white and gray matter. Further, research is showing that MS alters more body systems and body chemistry than previously recognized. A researcher writing in *Neurological Research* in 2006 summed it up: "Indeed, we know now that MS is not a purely demyelinating disease but a whole brain disease. The vastness of the pathology in MS and the fact that several pathogenic mechanisms work in concert have made a 'cure' for MS as yet unattainable."

Can We Come Together?

In some ways, the dietary approach and allopathic medicine are coming together. Allopathic medical studies have confirmed that omega-3 oil supplementation is beneficial and that vitamin D is helpful in prevention of MS—two tenets long held by the dietary treatment proponents. Other recent studies revisit molecular mimicry and Swank's focus on the blood-brain barrier. The newest drug, Tysabri, operates on the idea that if the activated immune cells do not cross the blood-brain barrier, then the disease mechanism is greatly reduced. That is very similar to the Recovery Diet's tenet that if the immune cells are not activated by an antigen (food), then they do not cross the blood-brain barrier and the disease process is stopped.

True to their empirical base, medical professionals point out that there are no studies to show that diet can make a difference in MS. It is important to clarify that no comprehensive studies have been done on the diet approach—so it has not been shown to be ineffective either. No institution with sufficient financial resources to be able to do such a large study has shown any interest in truly researching the dietary approach in its entirety. Even undertaking that study is a daunting task with the need for a research design that captures and tracks the many variables in the individual treatment programs.

While allopathic medicine continues to search for a complete understanding and cure, we assert that the Recovery Diet can help people now. The proponents of the diet approach use the science and research of allopathic medicine to augment our understanding of what works and why. In turn, allopathic medicine might learn from those of us who have beaten the disease through diet. Combining our knowledge can only help alleviate all the suffering that MS brings.

Let's work together.

4

Re-Membering the Body: The Benefits of Exercise

If we could give every individual the right amount of nourishment and exercise, not too little and not too much, we would have found the safest way to health.

—HIPPOCRATES

This basic truth about the necessity of right diet and right exercise for good health has been around for a long time. In the earlier chapters we have explained the complexity of MS, the proper diet for recovery, and the science behind it. This chapter is about the right exercise program and the basic concepts behind it to help you further your recovery process. The mysterious presentation of MS symptoms that are unique to you will benefit from the appropriate regimen.

It doesn't matter if the disease has robbed you of your ability to feed yourself, put you in a wheelchair for the last four years, or if you are in complete remission from a single MS exacerbation. We will outline the basic concepts of exercise and describe explicit exercises for you to do no matter what your level of function and mobility. You will learn how to re-member your body, putting all of your physical members back together so that you can function with a whole body once more.

Compromised neuromuscular responses will improve if you are willing to work at regaining them.

MS—Your New Exercise Partner

If you have been exercise-phobic in the past, having MS is a demanding and unpleasant new partner to work with. The chances that you will get worse if you don't change your habits—with food and with exercise—are prompting you to start taking these disciplines seriously. The good news is that it is never too late to begin. Science has shown that getting a good workout every day for the rest of your life will actually extend your life, as well as improve its quality. So start now because you have to and keep at it because you want to keep feeling better and more alive.

We now know that abandoning the Paleolithic diet has affected our modern bodies. It is important to know that ancient humans were designed for an active hunter/gatherer existence in order to get that food. Our ancestors were always on the move, eating when there was abundant food, and fasting when there was little available. Our metabolisms slowed down during the cold months or during a drought, conserving our energy for spring, when food would be ready for the taking once again.

Whether our modern lifestyles are afflicted by sitting in offices all day or by ill health, we are signaling our bodies to shut down, as if we were fasting for the long, lean months ahead. Chemicals for rebuilding the body slow down. Debilitating as our disease is, we contribute to that decline when we don't make any effort to move within our new limitations. Low energy resources will keep the basic core functions going, but there is nothing extra to spend on healing. Exercising at an appropriate level for you is therefore vitally important to accompany your diet changes. It signals your body that you are remembering how to be a modern hunter/gatherer again. It signals chemicals to start rebuilding the body to gear up for the active life ahead.

Regular exercise will help you to keep your muscle strength and tone, as well as keep your nervous system firing on all levels. As soon as you begin an exercise routine, you will be establishing a baseline for observation as you gain in balance, strength, and endurance. You can use these exercises to see which side of your body is weaker and which muscles you have been using to compensate. You will enjoy seeing how much you improve doing any particular exercise. The real payoff will be the functional improvement in your everyday life. When you can achieve rolling over in bed for the first time in a long while, or are out of your wheelchair and walking across the room, or biking for an extra mile with ease, then you will know just how beneficial exercise can be.

Body Attitude

The mind-set of a crippled person is as limiting as the person's body movements. Our sense of self is deeply entangled in our physical persona. The documentary film *Murderball* tracks male paraplegics and quadriplegics playing a Paralympic sport called murder ball, or wheelchair rugby. In it, these men came to terms with their disabilities and how passionately engaged with their bodies they became through this sport. Getting over the sense of being a victim is always the first step. Our thought processes are intimately linked with our bodies and finding the will to move on is necessary to start exercising.

People with MS react differently to the myriad ways of being affected by this illness. Sexual dysfunction (not achieving orgasm) is very demoralizing for some; bathroom anxiety (the urgency to urinate, the inability to release) is horrifying for others; simply using a cane or the need for a wheelchair feels like the end of life for still others. We all respond differently, and for you the overall exhaustion, the multisystem failure, could be the worst symptom of all.

You may need to shift your attitude as to what you can expect from your body during the process of healing. Keep in mind that having a gratifying sexual experience isn't only about achieving orgasm. Canes and disability stickers on your car are not the end of the world. Please discuss your concerns about any of these with your doctor, who may recommend a physical therapist, occupational therapist, or counselor for your specific needs. A physical therapist, for instance, can explain appropriate muscular exercises for recovering those more intimate functions not explained here. Although there are drugs to help with all of these symptoms, as you recover, you can look forward to eliminating them over time as you regain control over your own body by following the Recovery Diet.

People who care about you may volunteer to get you started in sharing what they do for exercise—yoga, Pilates, water aerobics, swimming, Alexander Technique, Feldenkrais, Continuum. Or join a gym with a knowledgeable sports medicine trainer. There are many kinds of massage and so many more practices to choose from. (See Appendix B for brief explanations about these healing movement practices.) If you live in a rural area with no exercise facilities or movement classes readily available, you can rent exercise videos and adapt them to your own needs, in your own time. Find an indoor swimming pool to build up strength moving against water resistance. Also, you cannot overheat in the water, and it helps support your body weight while you move.

Rewiring the Brain

MS has damaged the wiring throughout different parts of our brains. Axons have died, myelin sheathing has been destroyed and replaced with scar tissue, and systems feeding our brains have been compromised. Every movement we make happens through complex chemical interactions, which make the kind of electrical connections we need for every one of our muscles to move.

The brain, being the grand master of the entire body, has been granted many ways to circumvent disaster caused by trauma to itself. If the main highway is blocked by a rockfall, the messages are sent through a detour to arrive at the same or similar destination. For example, if the body has lost strength in the legs and pelvis, then the shoulders will gradually be told to take up the lost stability in walking, and become the compensating stabilizing force. You may have relearned how to walk by tightening your shoulders. (Relax your shoulders right now as you read this and see if they drop down a notch.) It is amazing how the brain tells the body to reorganize in order to keep on going.

How did we learn to move our hands in the first place? Babies come into this terrestrial world as watery beings. Water was where we first began as a species and where every cell in our bodies first formed inside our mothers' wombs. Infants' movements are wavy and unfocused. They bat ineffectually at objects that attract their attention for many weeks. At around four to five months old, a previously accidental hand in the mouth becomes a deliberate movement for the first time.

In baby brains the neurons, or nerve cells, have unattached branches that get hooked up together after repeated use. Complete circuits are created and thereafter used whenever the same movement is ordered to occur. The oligodendrocytes are called into action to make myelin sheathing, and that original message path becomes a superhighway coated with new fatty insulation. If circuits are not used often enough in the developing brain, the potential connections are washed away with a chemical solvent. Energy is not wasted to maintain what is no longer useful.

Repeated movements, or exercises, are what make these circuits complete. Neuroscience (brain research) has discovered that this process is not over once we grow up. As adults, the exact same process of wiring neurons together can take place again. The master of the body very much wants to find its way around its damaged roads, and given a chance, will build new circuits necessary for neuromuscular messages to take place. Researchers have discovered that people with MS who are asked to accomplish a simple movement use more cerebral brain circuits than people without MS doing the same task. That is, people with MS must think their way through a movement, whereas those who don't have MS will only use the motor section of the brain required.

This thinking our way across the room is not bad—it is a sign that we have many unused neurons ready to do whatever it takes to get us back to moving again. It may be a while since you were able to take your body for granted; for example, you don't have to think about walking on uneven ground. Using our brains to exercise is where we can begin. Our thinking mind becomes our ally to harness the creative genius of the brain to heal itself in the affected areas.

Your neurons need to be reconnected with one another. Exercise rebuilds this circuitry over time and with repetition. Repetitive movements built the original neuromuscular connections we made in the beginning of our lives. We can rebuild these connections as adults.

MS Exercise Pointers

You may have experienced a neurologist asking you to stand with your feet close together with your eyes closed. This is called Romberg's sign, and if you lose your balance, it is a good indicator that your *proprioceptive* functions have been compromised by MS. Proprioceptive functions tell us where we are in relationship to gravity and the space around us. It is a crucial function in maintaining balance and in calibrating how much effort we need to make in moving our bodies. If your eyes seem very tired at night, it may be because you are using your eyes to let you know where your body is all of the time. Small muscles in your legs and feet may have stopped giving you that feedback. Your eyes will take up the slack for as long as those feedback mechanisms are compromised. Proprioceptive exercises are included here, including safely working on variations of Romberg's sign until you have reclaimed this function.

Another specific tool to use is *visualization*. For those of you who are limited in your movements, this is where you will begin to move again. If you are in a wheelchair, you will start by visualizing yourself walking.

Just as athletes "see" themselves pole-vaulting over the bar an extra inch higher, crossing the finish line another two seconds faster, performing the triple axel jump on skates with greater ease before they take off, you can also use the power of visualization. Again, the mind is your ally, not your enemy when it comes to regaining lost control.

The trillions of neurons in our brain need to be reminded how to work and what to do as we re-member. New ones may also be called in to replace the work of those previously damaged. Think of what you want to move, visualize it happening, and try to accomplish that goal just a little. People who have had strokes have recovered the use of their weaker side by tying their stronger arm to their body and making the weaker one work no matter how clumsy it makes them feel. We all hate to be reminded of our weaknesses, but disciplined exertion should eventually have the desired effect.

Visualizing in a concentrated way literally stimulates the muscles to move. For this reason, visualizing exercises in this chapter before you attempt them will warm up the muscles before you begin. You can also visualize yourself accomplishing the exercises if you are unable to execute the movements because of physical compromise or fatigue, lack of space to move in, or you can mentally run through your routine in bed at night without waking your partner.

Simply *breathing more deeply* is also important. Our muscles need oxygen to do their work. If you know that your whole left side is more compromised than your right—that includes your left lung. Your diaphragm doesn't drop down as fully on the left side when you inhale. This affects your internal organs. Increasing your breathing is important, and visualizing the left lung working as hard as the right will help. By stimulating awareness of your lung through deep breathing you are letting awakening neurons know that this is another area that needs their attention. We have as many neurons as there are stars in the Milky Way. That means there are lots of potential partners to help you heal and relearn how to rebuild new movement circuits.

If you begin to feel sensation returning to your fingers, hands, and arms, you must give yourself many weeks to turn those feelings into muscular obedience, just as you did once before. You may also be someone who can easily articulate your fingers or other parts of your body but cannot actually feel the movement yet. Keep up the exercises, and for you, it may be sensation that needs healing time to return, rather than the movement itself.

Following in Our Own Baby Steps

Many therapeutic bodywork practitioners use the practice of replicating baby/toddler skills as a way to learn to stand and walk again. The developmental exercises that follow begin where we all began. First we use our eyes to track the world around us, which leads to rolling over. Then we proceed to crawling, sitting, standing, pulling up, and finally walking. Those of you who have serious limitations will spend a great deal of time doing this set of exercises.

Even if you are able to chase children around the playground, try these exercises as described. They will lay a good foundation for the more strenuous muscle-specific routines that follow. They will also give you a chance to slow down and rediscover the sensuous delight of basic movement. Babies have an inner mandate to become a fully functional bipedal human being as they push through into each stage. But they also revel in the sheer delight of experimentation until they discover what works best. Give yourself time to identify exactly where you are strong and where you are weak. Breathe, slow down, and enjoy the delight of moving for better health.

MS Movement Particulars

Unusual cycles of *rest and recovery* are another attribute of the MS body. It takes much longer for the heartbeat of someone with MS to slow down after vigorous exercise than for someone without MS. People with MS often sweat longer after getting overheated during a workout. It also takes longer to get feedback from your body to know when you have gone beyond your limit. This can be dangerous. You may be able to ski down a difficult slope, only to collapse suddenly when the physical stress is over.

The key is to slow down and deliberately rest after each exercise. Use the time to do a slow inside-body scan, head to toe, and breathe deeply. Open your attention to the more subtle signals that the mind will override if it is merely counting repetitions. Breathing consciously can help relax your muscles into a more willing state of cooperation, rather than pushing them too far, too fast.

Keep your own need for more rest stops in mind if you have a new bodywork teacher. You must be the one to tell your trainer when you must stop. A fast-paced aerobic-style exercise class could actually harm you, not help you heal. By taking things slowly and deliberately, you will be the one to know when to try something more challenging in terms of strength or endurance. Your responses are unique. Exercises must also be uniquely tailored for your body's abilities. All of us, not just people with MS, have inherent weaknesses and strengths. So choose a trainer wisely.

Another challenge to exercising is *pain*. If you have chronic pain in muscles or joints, then you must be careful about how you move. If your pain is caused by inflammation in a muscle, then your inclination is to stretch that muscle out because it feels so tight. The tightness from inflammation, however, is caused by fluid accumulating around sore tissue, not from a shortened muscle. In fact, shortening the muscle may actually bring relief and restore needed circulation again. Stretching out or lengthening the muscle may aggravate it. Knowing how to shorten a given muscle is something a trained bodywork professional can teach you.

Pain in a joint or muscle can be soothed by icing it for twenty minutes at a time. Although NSAIDs (nonsteroidal anti-inflammatory drugs such as aspirin, Aleve, or ibuprofen) aren't very good for you in the long run, as heavy use can damage your digestive tract, they can temporarily head off an inflammatory response if you sense you have overdone some activity, and allow more freedom of movement while preventing the usual inflammatory response. Breathing deeply in slow-moving yoga postures may be a good form of movement to explore.

If your pain is due to inflamed nerves present in some cases of MS, it is a far more mysterious and difficult issue to control. Inflamed nerves hurt, and it is exhausting and debilitating to endure without calming support. Mindfulness meditation, developed by Jon Kabat-Zinn from an ancient practice, has been used for pain control for many chronically painful conditions. It is even taught in some hospitals, as it has been shown effective in restoring a much-needed peaceful quality of life to those who suffer ongoing pain. See if you can find a teacher, a book, or online information about this practice for learning a new way to achieve pain relief.

If you are someone who suffers from MS discomfort, notice the ebb and flow of "constant" pain and take advantage of a good minute, hour, or day to try some gentle stretching exercises. You cannot actually harm yourself through movement if you have inflamed nerves. It is not dangerous to move unless the muscles are in spasm because of what is called "referred" pain.

It is essential at some point to have a trained professional advise you how to work safely and specifically on your body. Words in this book are not enough. Proceed safely, please!

The Exercises

Rolling Over

Rolling over is the first whole-body skill babies at around five months of age seem to accomplish. When you can roll over in bed on your own, this will signal the return of independent movement for you.

STARTING POSITION

Lie on your back. Let your eyes move very slowly all the way to the left. Take note of everything in your line of vision. Let the weight of your head follow your eyes and see if the gentle twisting of your upper spine leads to an urge to keep on rolling in that direction. This can take up to one minute.

THE WORK

Visualize rolling over onto your stomach when your head is turned as far as it can go, and encourage the influx of new imagined sensations. Hold this picture for at least ninety seconds. Slowly return your head to center until your eyes look straight up. Now repeat this entire process on the right side.

Increase the number of times you turn your head every day until you feel ready to attempt that roll. Having someone there to assist you *very gently* is also good at first. You may also need help getting onto your back once again to repeat rolling over on the opposite side.

THE GOAL

Keep practicing on your own until you can roll over, back and forth on both sides, with less and less effort.

Crawling

The alternating movement of left/right coordination of arms and legs while crawling like a four-legged mammal is a precursor to the upright bipedal motions of walking as a human being. It doesn't require the same relationship to gravity as standing up but still strengthens the muscles along the spine in preparation for standing. Also, you won't have far to fall if your arms and legs get tired.

STARTING POSITION

Lie on your back on a carpeted surface. Visualize yourself on all fours. Roll over onto your stomach and pull your hands in toward your body until your palms are beneath your shoulders. Push your upper body up and then push yourself backward up onto bent knees. Now you are on all fours. Check to see if you can feel your weight distributed evenly down all four pillars of arms and legs onto the floor, like a wobbly newborn colt. *Breathe.*

THE WORK

Drag the left knee forward several inches. Drag the right knee forward an equal number of inches. Rebalance on all fours. Shift the left hand forward several inches. Shift the right hand forward several inches. *Breathe.* Repeat this sequence if you can, several times.

THE GOAL

Eventually, shift the left knee and right hand forward at the same time. Shift the right knee and left hand forward at the same time. Practice lifting your limbs slightly with each knee and hand movement. This is crawling and an absolutely major step toward walking again. Practice crawling around for up to fifteen minutes at a time whenever you can. Be careful of your knees—if they start aching, stop immediately and lie down and stretch your legs out to rest them. Wearing knee pads that carpenters use may help.

VARIATION

Scrubbing a floor works (yes, Cinderella!) to get you to shift your weight and utilize many muscles in your trunk in order to stabilize your balance while you are working with one hand or arm. Try to scrub with the weaker side as well. Of course, you don't actually have to clean anything, but the circular movements in the upper body will call on your trunk muscles to hold you steady while you "scrub" clockwise and counterclockwise, using first one hand and then the other. Crawl forward or backward a few feet in between each scrubbing location.

Pulling Upright to Standing from the Floor

Pulling yourself up is the next step. If you haven't been upright out of a wheelchair in a while and bearing your own weight, you must take this very gradually. If you are regaining sensation in your back and feet and legs, it is time to harness these feelings into actual muscular function. You must have something strong enough for you to pull up on and someone nearby to spot you and help you get into a comfortable position again if you cannot get out of a tangle by yourself. Toddlers have it easy because the chair and the coffee table are just the right height for them to reach.

STARTING POSITION

On all fours, crawl next to a couch or sturdy chair or counter or windowsill that won't move if you pull on it. Visualize yourself pulling up to standing.

THE WORK

First, use the couch arm to pull yourself up halfway using both arms and hands. Next, use the taller couch back, or a chair placed next to a tall bureau, or a windowsill, and then perhaps a column in your living room to pull yourself all the way up to standing. Relax your upper body and focus on letting your legs and feet hold you up. Breathing as deeply as you can is important. Your muscles need oxygen to work at their optimal capacity. Practice letting your hands go gradually, transitioning with just barely touching the tips of the fingers to your support. Stand for thirty seconds, then lower yourself to the floor very carefully.

THE GOAL

Try standing up from the floor, holding on to the couch back for up to a minute, then two minutes, then up to five minutes at a time. Use your legs and feet more and more and your arms and upper body strength less and less to get up there. Lower yourself back down. Try this once a day, then twice a day, then up to 4 or 5 times in a row until you feel fairly fluid in your rising up and lowering down.

Proprioceptive Standing and Balancing

The next step is to find your balance standing up without clutching on to a support without using your eyes, relying on your own proprioceptive functions to know where you are in space.

STARTING POSITION

Stand with both hands on the edge of the kitchen sink. Close your eyes. Breathe deeply and retrain your feet to do the work of telling your body when it is in balance. Also try to shrug and relax your shoulders.

THE WORK

Gradually loosen your grip on the edge of the sink. If you are able to balance with your hands only lightly touching the sink, try doing it with just four fingers of each hand touching. If you can do that, then try just three, then two, then one finger, and then none.

THE GOAL

If you keep your hands hovering over the sink, you can catch yourself if you start to fall. Eventually, gradually increasing the time, you will be able to stand very still with your eyes closed for at least a minute without holding on.

VARIATION

You can also increase your proprioceptive awareness of one leg or the other by lifting one foot just off the ground while holding on to the edge of the sink. To begin, keep your eyes open. Increase the height of lifting one foot just a little bit every week. Decrease the number of fingers supporting you as above, until you are just hovering to catch yourself if necessary while balancing on one leg or the other. Beware of twisting your body when lifting either foot off the ground. Eventually, repeat the entire process with your eyes closed.

Trunk Muscles 1

Sitting up in a chair may be the necessary next piece for you. It may be that your legs are strong enough but you cannot lift up and out of a slumping posture. You would benefit from doing the following exercises every day. Sitting up without struggle will become as automatic as breathing.

STARTING POSITION

Lie on your back on the floor with your legs bent and your calves up on the seat of the couch (or chair or bed of the right height), your arms stretched out behind you. Breathe deeply and visualize your stomach and back muscles working while you move your legs independently, just as if you were walking.

THE WORK

Slide your right foot, dragging your heel across the cushion, toward the edge of the couch. Slide it back again. Repeat with the left foot. Gradually increase your repetitions up to 10 times on each side.

THE GOAL

Feel how your back and stomach muscles are activated in order to extend your limbs. Touch your lower back and belly with your hands to increase receiving feedback from those working muscles as you slide your legs back and forth.

VARIATION

Repeat with just the right arm down by your side, the other arm behind you. Repeat with just your left arm down by your side. This exercise may not be hard for many of you to do, but it is more about tuning in to the feeling of the internal experience of your trunk muscles working than it is about the moving of your legs.

Trunk Muscles 2

STARTING POSITION

Lie on your stomach on a mat or a rug with your arms extended out straight beyond your head. Visualize one leg at a time lifting slightly off the floor. Breathe deeply.

THE WORK

Lift your left thigh bone inside of your leg while keeping the muscle on the floor. Or imagine lifting it just high enough to slip a piece of paper under it. Return it to the floor. Breathe. Lift the right leg in the same way. Return it to the floor and relax and breathe.

THE GOAL

Feel how your back and stomach muscles tighten as you extend your legs prior to lifting them. This is using the trunk muscles so that sitting up and eventually your walking will be properly supported. Hold the lift for at least ninety seconds at a time. Repeat until you can do it up to 10 times on each side lifting your legs up to a couple of inches off the floor.

VARIATION

Instead of extending both arms beyond your head on the floor, bring your right arm down to your side while you lift the right leg. Return the leg to the floor and try the other diagonal using the left arm down and lifting the left leg. This works different muscle groups across the back and abdominal trunk muscles. Final variation is lifting both legs at the same time. *Caution:* Make sure you are pressing your pubic bone down into the floor as you try this. If you have lower back pain, this may put too much strain on your back. Strengthening your abdominal muscles must come first. See a physical therapist or a Pilates instructor to address this weakness before attempting to raise both legs.

Trunk Muscles 3

This addresses the many different abdominal muscles working in front of your trunk. Do this very slowly. As with many exercises, doing this once slowly and correctly is better than doing it superficially with speedy repetitions.

STARTING POSITION

Lie on your back on the floor and breathe in deeply. As you exhale, lift your head and shoulders to look down at your feet.

THE WORK

Place your hands on your abdominal area, first on the front, then on the sides as you practice this strengthening exercise. It is important to let your head and shoulders "float" up—let your belly do the work. The following visualizations will wake up those belly muscles. Imagine there are ropes attached to your pubic bone and you are pulling up on them. Imagine the string of your sweatpants tightening around your waist. Your sides will pull into a V shape funneling down to the width of your pelvic bones. Slowly return your head and shoulders to the floor using the same ropes and string to control your descent. Relax completely. Repeat every day until you can do this exercise slowly and smoothly 10 times.

THE GOAL

Again, this isn't about the raising of your head and shoulders, it is about harnessing the abdominal muscles. Your hands and fingers may tell you when those muscles are engaged before you can "feel" them working from the inside out. Having trunk support leads to being able to use the support of a walker even if your legs and feet are still numb and shuffling. Eventually, a cane will support your balance as a "third leg" for a tripod effect.

Conclusion of Developmental Exercises

This concludes the section of exercises following the developmental path we all once learned as young children. If you can roll over, crawl, sit, pull up to standing, and balance yourself with your own proprioceptive functions, and are walking with or without aids, the following exercises are designed to strengthen specific muscle groups you will need as you move about your daily life. There are many more muscle groups to explore than have been included in the following exercises. For instance, running along the outside of the legs are the external rotator muscles that supply the stability to walk in a straight line. As you progress and recover, you may want to seek out exercises beyond the scope of what is offered here.

Exercises for Specific Muscle Groups

Feet and Ankles 1

STARTING POSITION

Sit up in a straight-backed chair. Breathe and visualize your feet and toes, tops and bottoms, working at top capacity, strong and flexible with every step.

THE WORK

Curl the toes on your right foot upward. Point them down. Repeat on the left side. Keep breathing and keep your upper body relaxed. Shrug your shoulders to be sure they are not doing the job for your feet. Repeat 5–10 times on each side.

THE GOAL

The stronger your feet are, the better they will work when you are walking. Those of us who have experienced foot drop should notice definite improvement over time as the diet works to decrease symptoms and restore sensation and strength.

VARIATION

Tap your left foot up and down as quickly as you can. Tap your right foot in the same way. Notice which side is stronger or more responsive. Keep breathing and see if you can get both feet to tap at the same rate over a period of days, or weeks.

Trunk Muscles

STARTING POSITION

Sitting in a straight-backed chair, breathe and place you hands low down on your belly.

THE WORK

Lift your right foot just off the floor. Feel the pull down low in your abdominal muscles, somewhere in your groin area. Replace your foot on the ground. Repeat on the left side. Relax.

THE GOAL

Gradually increase the height when lifting your foot off the ground, taking weeks until you can lift your knees, one at a time, to waist height. Notice which side is stronger and visualize the weaker side lifting just as high without letting your trunk muscles cave in to do it. *Do not* lift any higher than your belly muscles can support you. Keep your back straight up and down, no twisting your spine in any way. Patience. Gradual. Breathe.

Feet and Ankles 2

STARTING POSITION

Lie on your back with your feet up against a wall and your knees bent. It's fine if you need to use big pillows or an exercise ball or box to support your thighs so that you can concentrate on your feet up on the wall. If you have trouble holding your legs parallel to each other, and your knees want to flop apart, you can use a quick release strap or tie a stretchy Thera-Band or Tigaband or belt around your thighs to keep your knees at a constant distance apart.

THE WORK

Slide the right foot up the wall as far as you can, keeping the sole of the foot in contact with the wall, leading with the toes. Slide it back down again to your starting point, leading with the heel. Repeat on the left side. "Walk" up and down up to 10 times on each side. Keep breathing, rest your legs on the floor, and relax completely when you are done.

THE GOAL

Articulating the feet is essential to recovering a smooth gait while walking. The stronger they are, the faster they will respond to walking on uneven ground or help you recover if you should trip. Your trunk muscles are also working in tandem with your feet. Check them out with your hands.

VARIATION

Instead of straight up and down, mark a diagonal line first to the left with the left foot (toward 10:00) and come back to center, then to the right (toward 2:00) with your right foot. Or, mark half-circles (from 12:00 to 6:00 and back again) with your big toe inscribing the path your foot will take, arcing down clockwise and then up counterclockwise, first using the right foot, then again with the left. Bring your legs down to the floor and relax completely when you are done.

Feet and Ankles 3

STARTING POSITION

Sit with your back against the wall, legs straight out in front of you. Breathe and visualize happy feet dancing for pleasure.

THE WORK

Point your toes on both feet down toward the floor. Flex them back up with your toes pointing up toward the ceiling. Breathe deeply and do this 5 times. Point and flex.

THE GOAL

Having independent movement of your left and right foot will increase your balance while walking. Getting each foot to become stronger will lead to increased balance with every step, allowing you to walk faster, with a smoother gait.

VARIATION

Alternate with one foot pointing down and the other foot in a flexed position with your toes straight up. Do it with straight legs 5 times each. Then when you flex one foot, bend your knee and slide the heel of your foot 12 inches or so toward your bottom. Keep the other leg straight with pointed toes down to the floor. Slide the bent knee down and point your foot while sliding the other heel in with flexed foot and bent knee. Use your belly muscles (use your hands to help locate them) to draw your legs in and out. Relax completely when finished and breathe throughout.

Exercise Balls

For those of you who are able to use them safely, I suggest getting an exercise ball. These balls are sold in many exercise and athletic stores and catalogues. They come in different sizes and can have more or less air in them for a squishy or bouncier feel. There are many brands. Get help from a salesperson to find which size is right for you. You should be able to sit on one with your feet comfortably flat on the floor.

Different sizes can be used for different kinds of exploration, such as a whole-body workout or isolating specific muscle groups. Many balls are sold with workout suggestions and you can adapt them to work safely for you. One safety measure is to always work on a soft carpet or mat, and another is to exercise in a corner so you have a wall on both sides nearby to catch yourself if you should start to roll off.

Spinal Flex

STARTING POSITION

Sit on the ball; your knees should be comfortably bent and your feet flat on the floor. Breathe.

THE WORK

Start a gentle bouncing movement, up and down. Feel the triangle that your big toe, pinkie toe, and heel make on the floor as you do so. Make your feet flat like a pancake and keep bouncing and breathing.

THE GOAL

The bouncing movement will start a gentle wave motion up and down your spine, waking it up from top to bottom. It is important to keep your shoulders relaxed. Small muscles in your feet, ankles, and legs will be rhythmically called into action as you bounce, thereby strengthening them for walking with a smooth gait. Try rolling your head around in a circle first to the right, and then to the left and keep bouncing. Shrug your shoulders up and down. Eventually, you should be able to bounce hard enough so that you are out of breath, establishing a gentle aerobic benefit.

VARIATION 1

Lie over the ball on your stomach. Let yourself breathe and roll around a little. Let your arms and hands dangle down in front of you, touching the floor as you roll forward, or with your legs and feet reaching to the floor behind you, stretching to balance as you roll backward. Roll side to side, and around in all directions. Breathe.

VARIATION 2

Sit upright on the ball, feet on the floor, and roll the ball with your bottom around in all directions. Breathe deeply. Bend forward with your hands on or near the floor, widen the position of your feet if you can, and continue rolling in wider and wider circles clockwise and counterclockwise. Feel the shifting stretches in your legs and back.

VARIATION 3

If your back is strong and your balance is already pretty good, try lying on your back over the ball. One suggestion, to be careful, is to clasp your hands together behind your neck as you stretch out over the ball on your back. Don't reach out behind you with extended arms or you may hurt your shoulders. Your legs and feet must already be strong enough to hold your weight so you don't slide down to your bottom too hard or roll off to one side. Roll the ball toward and away from your anchoring feet. Breathe deeply, especially into your back muscles.

Losing your upright position is very disorienting if your proprioceptive functions are at all compromised. Plenty of people without MS cannot do this, so *do not attempt this if you feel at all uncertain*. If you feel able to do this one, when you are finished arching your back over the ball, always go over the ball on your stomach again to uncurl your spine in the opposite direction.

Muscles Small and Large

Arms and Hands

STARTING POSITION

Sit comfortably on the floor, on a chair, or on a ball in front of a table. Have an assortment of objects—squishy balls, soft pillows, buttons, stones, or shells—in front of you.

THE WORK

Keep breathing as you squeeze and release soft things or pick up small objects and put them into piles first with one hand and then the other.

THE GOAL

The aim of all of these variations is for you to strengthen both hands until they are equally strong, gain proprioception, and increase your endurance for using them for longer and longer periods of time.

VARIATION 1

Draw a picture. Write a lengthy letter out longhand with a pen or type one on a computer.

VARIATION 2

With your right hand, tap each finger several times against your thumb. Repeat on your left hand. Or place your forefinger on your nose and then move it away at arm's length and back again. Repeat on the other side.

Hamstrings 1

The hamstrings run up the back of your legs. You will feel them especially when you walk upstairs or uphill.

STARTING POSITION

Lie down on the floor on your stomach. Bend your arms with your palms flat on the floor about 12 inches in front of your shoulders.

THE WORK

Breathe. Push your upper body up off the floor, leaving your forearms flat on the ground and both hips squarely on the floor. Breathe and let your head "float" up, looking straight ahead. Bend your right leg at the knee, and bring your calf toward your bottom. Place it down gently. Repeat with the left leg.

THE GOAL

Working first with flexed feet, do some with pointed toes as well. If the movement is jerky and you can only lift your lower leg two inches off the floor, that is fine. Start where you are. Take it slowly day by day, until you can easily do 10 smooth up and downs with pointed and flexed feet on each side, able to almost kick yourself in the butt.

Hamstrings 2

If you are strong enough to work standing up, try this one.

STARTING POSITION

Stand facing a wall. Stand far enough away that you can extend your arms with your palms flat on the wall.

THE WORK

Without collapsing in your trunk at all, do a wall push-up. Bend your arms very slowly as your face comes toward the wall. Breathe. Straighten your arms again and do up to 10 push-ups.

THE GOAL

Again, this isn't so much about the strength in your arms as it is about feeling the connection of your hamstrings and your lower back and your abdominal muscles as you move toward the wall. Feel the release of those working elements as you push away.

Quadriceps

If you have ever skied, you probably already know this exercise. Your quad muscles run along the top of your thighs and you need them for walking, squatting, getting in and out of chairs, and especially walking uphill or climbing stairs.

STARTING POSITION

"Sit" against a wall with your knees slightly bent, your back flat on the wall. Your knees should be under your hips, your feet pointing straight ahead on the floor beneath your knees. Adjust your feet, if necessary, to the correct width.

THE WORK

Push down into your feet as if you were going to slide back up the wall, but stay put. Breathe and hold this for at least ninety seconds, more if you can. Slide back up, rest, and try it again.

THE GOAL

This should get you feeling your quads and strengthening them in no time. You may feel them all the way from the top of your thigh down to where they insert by your knees. If your knees ache after this, try to push the floor away harder with your feet. Build up over many days to lengthening the duration of this stretch.

Walking and Sports Goals

If you are already ambulatory, practice going up and down the stairs without holding on. If you can walk one block easily, try two next time.

Here is an exercise that most people with MS can use. The sides of our bodies are usually underutilized and they have a great deal to do with our proprioceptive functions and maintaining our balance.

STARTING POSITION

Stand parallel to a wall with your arms outstretched at shoulder height.

THE WORK

Step out with the right foot, bring the left foot in beside it and repeat, until you reach the end of the room. Return, leading out with the left foot.

THE GOAL

This exercise is about waking up the sides of the body and increasing your balance. You may be able to walk in a straight line without a problem but may find leading from the sides of your body to be more of a challenge. This will increase your proprioception and give you strength connecting the small muscles in your feet and ankles to the whole leg and the sides of your trunk muscles, preventing a fall should you trip or stumble.

If you are already hiking or doing any kind of active sport, note your endurance and beware of overdoing it. Always warm up gently before undertaking any activity. Find your limits realistically and only go beyond them in incremental installments to build up stamina. A gentle noncombative martial art like tai chi or aikido (more active, working with partners) may be worth looking into if you are searching for a different kind of workout. Try ballroom or other kinds of dancing. Be creative in your explorations as you get stronger muscularly and gain in endurance.

VARIATION

Try doing a crossover step with the left foot in front or then in back of the right as you move sideways. Then reverse it to return.

Rediscover the Joys of Childhood

If you ever feel discouraged, remember: Toddlers don't hate their bodies for being clumsy, and you were a toddler once. Toddlers are the most amazing scientists. They make constant hypotheses—"That looks like a shiny thing up there!"—and find a way to discover the engineering and physics necessary to reach that thing. Once toddlers have something in their hands, they ask, "Does it taste good?" Or they wonder, "Will it throw far?" They discover with abandoned delight whether something is harder or softer than "me," wetter or dryer than "me," taller or smaller than "me." They are in constant discovery mode. They want to swallow up the world they perceive around them as intensely as they can. They roll over, sit up, crawl, stand, and fall a lot before they conquer walking. You did that once and you can love your body again by giving it an educated chance to exercise daily in both small and committed ways.

Paying Attention

Paying more attention to how your body experiences movement is part of utilizing this diet. Knowing that particular foods are responsible for restoring your body, you will now pay more attention into both what goes into your body and what makes it feel better or worse and why. Exercising the body uses the same principles; knowing what makes you feel good—feel stronger, go on for longer, or experience more positive sensations—and why. Learn to love your body. People with MS seem either to be bitter or at peace with their lives and themselves. Being resentful can never help your body to heal. Having self-love means loving the body that you have; maybe consciously for the first time.

Paying attention to others with the same loving attention we give ourselves as we recover is a great gift that this Recovery Diet offers us.

Learning to pay attention in healthy ways increases our participation in life and with others. Why else are we here?

Judi had a client once who had ALS and was losing muscular control and sensation at an alarming rate. Judi taught her some Continuum basics and at the end of the session her client held up her dangling hand and said, "This gives me body hope." She could feel powerful sensations coursing through her arms and hands for the first time in a long while. We can be inspired by her and by all of us who are compromised and look for physical ways to give us body hope. With this diet, and with exercise, there is hope for you and others like us.

Our neurological deficits can bring us great rewards as we rewire our neurons to find new pathways to move again. Neuroscience now confirms that we do build innovative pathways as adults, despite neuronal destruction due to illness or trauma. As babies, we created superhighways of interconnection as we gained in repeated patterns of muscular control. Through constant repetition, we learned to pick up the Cheerio or, later on, to ski and ride bikes. We can now enjoy the benefits of exercising knowing that as we re-member to function as healthy active adults, we are rebuilding circuitry in our brains.

Paying more attention in a positive way to our bodies is paying more positive attention to our minds, and vice versa. They are inseparable. The body and the mind and the heart working together are an unbeatable team. Paying attention to life is a prescription for all of us, with or without MS, for a healthier life in every way.

5

Depression: A Block to Healing

Ruth, who is profiled in a later chapter and is still living symptom-free, called one day and said, "There should be a chapter on attitude. I'm beginning to think that it is everything—without the right attitude, a person would never follow the diet or take a positive approach to MS."

Ruth had just witnessed a fellow person with MS pass away. This particular man had not only lived in her town, but also had been diagnosed at the same time she was, with the same severity in their conditions. She had watched as he had gone downhill to the point of having to be in a nursing home, though still in his forties. Through the years since they had both been diagnosed, she had been concerned about him—his negative attitude toward trying anything to help himself, toward the disease, and toward life in general. She felt that it all contributed to his early death.

Not a Choice: A Prison

Being depressed is not a choice—it insidiously sneaks into a person, coloring his or her every thought and preventing action. If engulfed by the paralysis of depression, a person will view the Recovery Diet as an impossible feat because they can't find the energy or the interest to even begin. This pessimistic attitude will lock them in the predominant downward spiral of MS.

Though not everyone with MS becomes depressed, a significant number do, whether as a part of the disease process or as a result of the impact of the disease on a person's life. If you are vulnerable, we hope this chapter will help you avoid the trap of depression. As with multiple sclerosis, the battle against depression can be fought and won.

What Is Depression?

Everyone experiences ups and downs, which are part of life's experience. After a loss or a disappointment, there is most often a reaction of sadness or melancholy, a contemplative depression. All of this is normal and usually passes with time.

Major depression is an entirely different state, in which people are so overwhelmed and immersed in their feelings of sadness, emptiness, hopelessness, worthlessness, guilt, apathy, and despair, there is no other reality for them. Depressive symptoms also vary, usually manifesting as either extreme on a continuum such as either not eating or eating too much, not sleeping or sleeping too much. It is also marked by other sleep disturbances, like waking up in the middle of the night and being unable to get back to sleep. The person's cognitive abilities are often affected, with loss of concentration, increased irritation, agitation, and inability to think rationally. Also, a depressed person has little energy, or interest in anything, and can no longer get pleasure from activities. It is truly a debilitating state, in which suicidal thoughts often occur.

As in the general population, depression affects a significant number of people with MS from all walks of life and from diverse life experiences. Usually the cause—a life event or circumstance—can be identified and treatment given. Some people seem to be more prone to depression than others; whether this is due to genetics or the environment is unknown. People without this tendency can face horrendous tragedies, and though they may be sad or down, never experience the paralyzing blackness of a major depression. In contrast, people who are vulnerable find themselves deep in depression over what, to the casual observer, doesn't look like such a major challenge.

Treatment Options

The good news is that depression is treatable with psychotherapy, medication, or both. It is important for people with MS to seek treatment for their depression so they can get back their energy and motivation to recover. Under the influence of a full depressive episode, the person with MS does not have the interest, motivation, cognitive ability, energy, and desire to get better, allowing the disease to run rampant, taking over their life.

Medication

There are several families of antidepressant drugs that can be effective in lifting mood. Despite advertising to the contrary, the exact mechanism of these drugs is not clearly understood. Studies done with serotonin often cite deficiencies in that body chemical as the cause of depression. However, so far these have not proven a direct correlation between levels of serotonin in the body and depression. Something else, as yet unidentified, is going on that makes these drugs effective.

As there is not a clear criterion to determine which drug is effective for which person, due to a limited understanding of both the etiology of depression and the mechanism of the drugs, finding the right medication and dosage is a matter of trial and error. Often, you may need to try several different regimes before you find the right combination. Also note, antidepressants take up to several weeks to start alleviating symptoms, so some patience is required.

Once the right medication and dosage is determined, these medications can be very effective. After the depression passes, it is important to have medical supervision throughout and especially when going off any antidepressant, as there can be side effects from a hasty withdrawal.

Psychotherapy

Seeing a trained professional counselor can be as effective as taking medication, according to studies done on this issue. The relapse for patients on pills is higher than for those getting cognitive-behavioral psychotherapy.

Again, there is not an exact science to psychotherapy, so it is important to find a therapist who feels right to you. By this I mean finding a good match with someone whom you can relate to, who seems to have a good understanding of your problems, and whose interventions both make good sense and are helpful.

Framework of Depression

The following conceptual framework is very effective in helping people understand and therefore break the depressive cycle and mood. This framework includes the characteristics of depression and the cycle of depression.

Characteristics of Depression with MS

It is useful to understand the four main components of depression: loss, anger, guilt, and low self-esteem. A diagnosis of MS and certainly the challenge of living with the disease can generate all four of these feelings very easily. It is when they dominate your mind and energies that depression can take over.

Loss

There is the obvious loss of function, like being able to walk, see, lift, and fully do all that you could do before. Then there is the loss of energy and vitality that can dramatically alter what you can accomplish in a day.

On a more subtle level, you may feel a loss of trust in the body or in life in general. People with MS may not feel whole or safe in their world.

The feelings of loss in MS can go further when careers end and relationships are destroyed because of the disease. Our sense of identity is very often tied to "what we do" and we fear losing that sense of purpose and worth. Those with MS face change and possible loss in their relationships because sometimes those close to them can't make the transition or feel comfortable in the presence of someone with a chronic disease. They also may flee the ill-suiting role of caretaker.

Anger

Anger is the understandable, even predictable, consequence of loss. It can be directed at the self, the body, the unfairness of life, the culture that marginalizes people with disability, or at fate, bad luck, or the divine.

Anger can also be used as a defense against the feeling of helplessness, aloneness, inferiority, and just plain being stuck. Anger is often the public face of depression—people sometimes prefer to hold on to rage to block out the blackness of depression.

It can also be the face of envy. Watching others, whom we perceive as perfect and whole, angers us as we are humiliated by daily stumbles. Rather than deal with our own feelings, it is often those we envy who bear the brunt of our emotions.

Guilt

This sneaky emotion that eats away at a person's insides often remains unnamed and unacknowledged. Blame accompanies guilt, each activating the other. Guilt and blame are pervasive in our culture; we blame the poor for their poverty, the sick for their illnesses, the parents for everything their children do, and the government for natural disasters, and this blame is often accepted and turned to guilt. In our common cultural view, there is a sense that we somehow caused and, worse, deserve our afflictions. What we get in life as a punishment or a reward is tied to our sense of being deserving or undeserving; in other words, guilt.

Loss of Self-esteem

In a culture that worships beauty, youth, and perfection in appearance, people who are less than perfect are eschewed, shunned, and ignored. The disfigured, the old, and the disabled often discomfit society because they are reminders that everyone is vulnerable to sickness, accident, and ultimately death. The message is clear: If you are imperfect, you are inferior.

Consider how this message affects our general population. Billions of dollars are spent on diet programs that promise a perfect body, plastic surgery to create beauty and youth, and exercise programs to sculpt the body to the desired long, lean form no matter what your bone structure. In comparison, much less money is spent to fix up the unseen aspects—our souls, our character, or our spiritual life.

It is only logical that people with MS may internalize this cultural value and norm along with everyone else. By this standard of perfection, just about anyone comes up short and people with MS find themselves especially lacking. Self-esteem suffers. Add to that the common judgment that the disease is somehow deserved or caused and self-esteem drops another notch.

As understandable as it is that depression oftentimes accompanies MS, the good news is that is doesn't have to be that way.

The Spiral of Depression

Another helpful way of looking at depression is understanding the self-perpetuating spiral of emotions that pulls a person deeper into despair. This leads logically to an understanding of the actions needed to reverse the spiral and climb out of the depths of depression. An illustration best shows this:

Feeling depressed

Doing less

Loss of good feeling about self

Lower self-esteem

Guilt

Anger at self for not doing more

Feeling inferior

Feeling more depressed

Guilt for feeling depressed

Lower self-esteem

Rage at world

Doing even less, crying or sleeping

Anger at self

Feeling like a big nothing; full of despair

By this illustration, it is clear that the continued judgments on self feed the depression until all sense of self-worth is destroyed. Suicidal ideation often results for the total loss of self-regard with the thinking pattern of "I am so worthless, everyone and the world would be better off without me here."

At its deepest, depression is paralyzing, leaving people with little to work with if they buy into all the usual thinking and values.

Out of the Depths

The first step in fighting depression is to reverse the spiral. Activity bestows good feelings about doing and being, though it takes great energy to get up and get out. Interactions with people in a positive way feed self-esteem. Good feelings bring more energy and with that more activity, pushing you back up the spiral.

The complaint of depressed people is that this all sounds good, but they don't have the energy to do anything. That may be true, but if they continue on the spiral, they will have even less. What is required, like swimming upstream, is to do, despite the lack of energy. A depressed person will say, "I feel better when I am out, it is just getting there that is so difficult." This is where courage and determination are needed—you have to fight for life. Much as in a war or a catastrophe, you have to dig down deep for the courage or just the desperate strength that can be drawn from the primal will to survive.

If you are feeling depressed, be patient and kind to yourself and start with small steps. One day, perhaps getting out of bed is all you'll be able to do. Another day, perhaps try a walk around the block or make a phone call to a friend. Each little step builds upon the previous one, and before too long you will start feeling better.

The importance of getting exercise and being out in the light, preferably sunlight, can't be underestimated. In some depressions, ultraviolet light is a highly effective treatment—this should be tested out if you suffer from depression. Exercise produces natural tranquilizers in the body, relieving depressed feelings.

Beliefs and Attitudes

Attitude springs from the very core beliefs that guide us through life. Whether we are aware of them or not in our daily lives, it is worth bringing them to consciousness and examining them. Our very core beliefs and the values we hold and live by come into play in all aspects of our lives, more than we may realize.

Two critical questions and how we answer them have tremendous influence on how we conduct our lives. The first: What is life about? The second: How do we measure the value of a person?

What Is Life About?

If people believe that, with a little work, they should have everything in life they want—the perfect career, the perfect spouse and family, and all the material goods—they are set up for trouble when problems arise. There is no place for adversity in this philosophy. A diagnosis of MS would be seen as unfair and unjust with the resulting anger, even rage that such a thing could happen. The narcissistic insult of a flawed body would be of immense proportion. The result of this kind of thinking would make the individual more vulnerable to depression. Often along with this life view is the sense of entitlement and power over their own life. MS shatters this illusion.

Many people internalize the teachings of a religion or spiritual practice. In most religions, suffering is seen as an integral part of life, challenging the person not only to endure, but to transcend their suffering. The goal is growth and drawing nearer to the divine, with suffering a vehicle to accomplish this. In this context MS is more acceptable, since the belief system holds that everyone is tested by suffering in some way, not always seen or evident to others.

M. Scott Peck, in his writings, observes that if you expect that life will be difficult at times, it is easier to both accept and deal with suffering. With this attitude, each of us is less likely to fall into the trap of self-pity and rage at the indignity of unfairness, and instead deal with what comes down life's path.

Try not to evaluate every life event as being bad or good. Each such judgment has a consequence in mood or attitude. The concept of deserving is also interesting and seductive, but ultimately doesn't really end in an answer. Sympathy, like self-pity, can be very appealing, but not constructive. Life is not conducted by a scale, or if there is one, it is beyond our comprehension. Bad things happen to good people.

It is much easier to maintain your spirits by seeing everything that happens as just life. As such, life is to be coped with, learned from, and in an odd way, no matter what aspect it presents, to be enjoyed for what it is.

How Do We Measure a Person?

Another crucial question that can make a difference in how we feel about our disease: What is valuable about any individual? If we take our cues from TV and magazines, our value comes from "what we do" and "how we look," that is, our careers, how much money we have, and, finally, our attractiveness. In the appearance category, being thin and fit, pretty or handsome, and well dressed and groomed are basic requirements. Youth, richness, and a certain level of dress and accessories add a premium. Under this grading system, MS can really lower our value in our own minds as well as in the minds of others.

However, if the size of a person's heart and the color of their soul—which refers to the virtues of charity, compassion, kindness, integrity, altruism, capacity to love, and lightness of spirit—are the yardsticks we use to measure a person, whether someone has MS or not has no effect. In fact, if having MS makes people more compassionate and charitable, then the disease has served a good purpose. In the long run it will increase those individuals' worth and perhaps raise their self-esteem.

To successfully live with MS, it is worth examining your very core beliefs. Even if they are out of daily consciousness, as they often are, they are still very powerful.

Walking the Line

There is a fine line between acceptance and determination to overcome the disease and giving up in resignation and raging against the disease. It is not an easy line to walk, but a positive attitude provides the best prognosis for recovery.

Acceptance is not giving up and allowing the disease to take over a person's life. It is saying that you acknowledge and, in an odd sense, honor the disease's presence in your life. It is giving up self-pity and any sense of hopelessness. Wallowing in those emotions has its unique appeal, like being a martyr. However, they all lead downhill.

It is also giving up the rage that MS happened to you, along with any sense of entitlement to a perfect life or other feelings about the unfairness of it all. It also means not allowing yourself to envy others' health and entertain fantasies of what you could do, if only.

These negative emotions rob you of needed energy, which could be better used in your recovery. Try to think, "Yes, my body has this disease mechanism or whatever it is, but I am going to minimize it so I can better coexist with the disease." In a sense, this approach takes away the disease's power to disrupt your life and gives it back to you to strengthen and affirm the health of your body. Negative emotions are corrosive, while a sense of power is affirming. Keeping a positive attitude is invaluable to your recovery.

6

Maintaining Your Recovery

Based on the experience of others who have followed the Recovery Diet over the last several years, you can expect to become symptom-free or at least have very minor residual symptoms. The process to your final end point will probably take years, though your symptoms will fade and healing will begin much earlier, which will enable you to return to a more normal life.

Healing

To get to the point where you are symptom-free and can begin to reintroduce foods to your diet, healing must take place in several body systems.

First, the disease activity must be stopped so that eating specific foods no longer triggers symptoms. With MS, it is always a balance between destruction and rebuilding, and when symptoms are no longer triggered, the body can go on healing, full speed ahead.

It has been shown that within the CNS, myelin is replaced and lesions can disappear. Nerve fibers can also be repaired or replaced, or new circuits created. The healing that takes place in the CNS is responsible for the return of lost functions and the elimination of altered sensations, as the correct messages can be sent from the brain to outlying limbs and body systems.

The breaches in the blood-brain barrier need to seal off so that, if and when the immune system is activated by allergens, illness, or stress, there is no leaking into the CNS. Autopsies have shown areas where the blood-brain barrier has healed, and the corresponding lesion became inactive.

Not only to prevent further MS attacks, but also for health in general, the digestive system needs to heal, so that the entire gut lining is healthy and protected by the beneficial microbes that aid in digestion. As your MS becomes inactive, watch for reactions like stomachaches, gassiness, nausea, or headaches, right after eating, as an early warning sign of some digestive problems.

Recovery from MS can go beyond being symptom-free and regaining all lost abilities and restoring full energy. It is also possible to add foods that were formerly restricted, after a certain amount of time passes and healing is done. The T cells can and do forget which foods were identified as foreign invaders. It has been shown that, over time, the immune system will stop activating to the introduction of former allergens. An example of this is seen in the ELISA and RAST tests. A food that was ingested just before the procedure and in a large quantity will produce a much higher reading on the scale than another food that was not ingested for a long time before the test date. If wheat has not been ingested for months or years, the immune system might not react at all, even though wheat formerly triggered major symptoms. Again, this depends very much on the individual, as you can expect with MS. In recovery, we take advantage of that fact.

However, in order not to reactivate the immune response, it is advisable to be prudent. The guideline from the rotation diet, used to help people get over their allergies, is not to eat any of the formerly offending foods more than once every four or five days. It is also important not to eat too large a quantity of these foods at any one time. Rotation and moderation are keys to continuing a successful recovery, but at the same time, enabling you to return to eating some of the former trigger foods.

When you are sufficiently recovered, you can test your different trigger foods to see if the immune system still reacts. If there are no adverse reactions or symptoms such as headaches or stomachaches after several [illegible] safe to assume that you can eat these foods [illegible]tion.

[illegible]king about MS, this is highly individualized. [illegible]n able to return to a normal, even a slightly [illegible]thers find there are some foods they can never [illegible]

[illegible] individual is the amount of time it takes to get to [illegible]Most people with MS are so grateful for the return [illegible]rgy that, whenever they reach this final stage, they [illegible]healing can take some time, but again, if the trend [illegible]g toward healing after years of being attacked by [illegible]tainly worth the wait.

Need for Care—Not a Cure

With symptoms gone, energy restored, and a return to normal eating, it is easy to think of yourself as cured. Wonderful as these results are, remember that the diet is not a cure.

The template that was laid down in your body for the sequence of events that characterize MS is still there. The genetic factor, the change in the immune system's ability to distinguish self-cells from outside antigens, the underlying vulnerability to breaches in the blood-brain barrier, and whatever other unknown factors that contribute to MS are probably still there. With full recovery and control, whether you are actually cured or not doesn't really matter.

A person may go along for years with no problems, lulled by normalcy. They become lax in health habits and eating. Then a day may come when they are jolted back to MS reality with the onset of a symptom.

The good news is, if MS activity does return, you can again stop, reverse, and recover through the same dietary means. But who wants to go through that twice? John Pageler, who recovered first under the guidance of Dr. Swank, went on a protracted binge of hamburgers, French fries, and milk shakes, only to find himself back in MS. He recovered once again through the diet, but time and energy were wasted.

Remember the Lessons Learned

It is better to be prudent and keep within the behaviors that maintain your recovery. People who have had MS might have to accept that they will always be a little fragile when it comes to health and act accordingly by taking good care of themselves. Actually, in our modern society, it would be good if everyone slowed down and took better care of themselves. We would all benefit in our national health, health-care costs, and general well-being as a nation.

Remember the lessons learned while actively recovering:

Listen to your body, respect it, and respond to it. A constant fatigue is often a precursor to MS's manifestation. Be aware if you are tired beyond what would normally be expected for your activities. Better yet, don't overextend yourself. Again, if you get a sick feeling after eating a particular food, it might be prudent to avoid it.

Get sufficient rest. Sleep is the time our bodies use to restore and heal from the wear and tear of life. With enough sleep, your body can stay ahead of the game, thus ensuring mental, emotional, and physical functioning at peak levels.

Exercise is always important. "Use it or lose it" is the expression. Man is a physical being whose body needs to be well used. During exercise, nerves fire, blood courses through our veins, and our digestion moves along quickly to supply our bodies the needed nutrients. Keep your body stronger than any disease.

Eat a healthy, well-balanced diet. Maintain sensitivity and awareness to all the subtle reactions of your body, as well as signs about any other aspect of life. Eat well and within the parameters that have proven to work for you.

Getting enough sunshine is important, even if you are heat sensitive. Skin cancer is a threat, but not receiving enough vitamin D coming in from our solar star is also detrimental to your health. Moderation is also called for in sun exposure, and getting sufficient vitamin D is now recognized as a real support for people with MS.

If You Have Difficulties

It is not understood why some people become totally symptom-free and, after time, can eat anything with impunity while other people's recoveries involve some residual symptoms and a continued need for a restricted diet. Factors such as the number and degree of food sensitivities, the ability of the body to heal, and the individual nature of the particular person all come into play.

John Pageler's newsletter was mailed to many hundreds of people who were following a more rudimentary diet approach. In it, he stated that you can recover as much as you want, indicating that the degree of your recovery is determined by how strictly and how long you stay disciplined. This may not be entirely true but is probably a factor.

A disease profile in which there are numerous offending foods, including all the "fillers," such that a person has a hard time eating enough to feel full, makes continued strict adherence to the diet difficult over time. It then becomes a matter of choices. In order to feel satisfied and not be hungry, the person might choose to live with a certain number of symptoms.

Another situation in which strictly adhering to the diet may not work is when there is a vast number of offending foods to which there are only subtle alterations of feelings—a faint feeling at most—and the person does not want to have to eliminate all of these minor triggers. In balance, it might be easier to live with the faint feelings than to become so strict as to limit the enjoyment of life.

In both of the above cases, the disease is controlled. A choice is made as to what level of recovery versus what level of strict adherence to a diet is most comfortable and works best for any particular person's life.

As anyone who has tried to lose and keep off excess pounds knows, it is not easy to maintain a diet. Witness to that difficulty is the recidivism rate—ninety percent—for weight losers. The stakes are much higher in maintaining recovery from MS, but it still is a test of willpower.

Human nature being what it is, and all of us being human, it is perfectly all right to choose a less than perfect recovery. The beauty of this is that it is under your control, not the control of the disease. The goal is to live a full, happy, and normal life.

Your Inner Self

Almost all people who have embarked on the Recovery Diet have spoken about what they learned on a personal and spiritual plane. One of the lessons of MS may be that it is what we are that counts, not what we do; we are human beings, not human doings. Whatever you take from your healing journey, honor and cherish it. This is not a smooth road, and the prize is not easily won.

Conclusion: Take Control of Your Health

The six chapters of Part 1 present all the knowledge, theory, research, tools, methods, and specific instructions to successfully discover and follow your Recovery Diet to a symptom-free life.

There is nothing in the diet that causes harm or any risk to health. On the contrary, it is expected that the general health of anyone following the diet will improve.

The diet does not counter any prescription. A person can be under medical care, take one of the CRAB drugs, and still pursue this treatment.

To embrace this diet is to embrace a new way of looking at health care. In the parlance of medical insurance, you can become your own "primary health-care provider." You can choose your own lifestyle, professional healing partners, and an entirely new relationship to your body.

PART 2
Stories of Healing

In Part 2, we offer you inspiring personal profiles of some who have reaped the benefits of the Recovery Diet. There are thousands who have fought this battle with MS and won. This book presents only a few. These are in sharp contrast to the well-documented cases of progressive disability caused by MS that are more commonly known and presented in the media.

7

...nn's Story

...997. As my husband and I waited in the wood-paneled examination room at the Mayo Clinic, settled in a pair of sturdy old leather chairs left over from a bygone era, I couldn't help thinking about all the sick people who had waited in this room over the years, just as we were, hoping and praying that they would find an answer to their health problems.

With one leg deadened and both feet lost to a strange numb/tingling sensation, I could barely hobble around. More and more often, I needed to hold on to someone in order to walk with confidence because there was no solid feeling in my feet. Worse yet, an all-encompassing fatigue had sapped me of energy and robbed me of any enjoyment of life.

Then, at odd and unpredictable times, I'd be struck with transitory symptoms including strange pains, tightness, and numbness, most often in my cheek or arms. Clearly, something horrible was happening to me, taking me on a downward slide. I was terrified.

So I sat there with my husband, waiting for the doctor to put a name to my condition and, of course, to cure me. The door opened and we instinctively straightened up as our senses quickened. The doctor, a sturdy middle-aged man, got right to the point: "You have multiple sclerosis." I burst into tears.

I knew enough about MS even then to understand that his words meant my ten months of agony were not going to end; rather, the destruction and erosion of my abilities had just begun. Multiple sclerosis, I knew, was a chronic, degenerative disease for which there was no cure, no escape. When I first went to the clinic for tests the week before with my oldest son, Edward, as my support, MS had been mentioned. And even before that, the neurosurgeon I'd seen had said the ominous words. But in the face of my tears, he had couched his potential diagnosis in enough "ifs" and "perhapses" that I had been able to dismiss the possibility. The power of denial being what it is, I had completely pushed those two words out of my mind, maintaining my ignorance.

Now, grasping for any way out of this sentence, I asked if maybe my ailment was just a cousin of MS. With a sad smile, the doctor told me the disease didn't have any cousins. Since my first major attack had occurred more than six months before, the usual steroid treatment would no longer be effective, he explained. Doctors, I've found, consider only dramatic changes that bring new persistent symptoms, which they call exacerbations, to be worth their attention. The protocol for a new exacerbation involves medicating the patient with strong steroids, such as prednisone, in order to reduce the inflammation. Since there is no way to measure and no help at all for the daily variations and transitory symptoms that so torment people with MS, doctors tend to ignore them and discourage any calls about this aspect of the disease.

At the time, the ABC drugs (Avonex, Betaseron, and Copaxone) had already been introduced, but the doctor at the Mayo Clinic did not mention them—for which I am now grateful. I am also glad that he didn't provide many details about the course of the disease and made no predictions for my future. Instead, his moist eyes met mine and he said simply, "Take care of yourself." When I tell people of this experience, they are stunned that he offered me no treatment or advice, thinking that he was somehow remiss in his duties. In truth, however, he did me a favor by not offering me anything more than that one sentence—and not leading me to believe that he had something effective to offer. Like most doctors, he did tell me to call if I had another major attack (or exacerbation), but not to call to discuss the daily changes or any symptoms that did not last for twenty-four hours.

My husband and I left the clinic that day stunned, defeated, and in despair, knowing that our lives were about to be irrevocably changed.

Multiple Sclerosis Attacks

About ten months earlier, the night before Halloween 1996, I had taken a strange fall. At that time I was forty-eight years old with two sons in college and a daughter in her sophomore year of high school. For most of my married life, I had worked part-time as a psychotherapist or as a college instructor teaching social work, but to help pay our children's tuitions I had just returned to work full-time as a therapist in a psychiatric clinic. Even though I had been very tired all that autumn, I had not slowed down, working full-time, going to weekend conferences or to visit my sons at college, attending my daughter's volleyball games and weekend tournaments—and that night attending a lecture. I remember being so exhausted that evening that I had briefly considered leaving before the program even started. In the end, I stayed, but when it was over, I rushed out. My legs felt very strange as I ran through the hall and down the few steps from the building, but, anxious to get home, I ignored them. Then, in the parking lot, down I went with such force that the wind was knocked out of me. Sprawled on the blacktop, I gasped for breath. Still, embarrassed by my clumsiness, I assured the people who rushed to help that I was fine, brushed myself off, and continued on my way to my car. I must have tripped.

The next morning, I not only had a huge bruise covering a good portion of the left side of my chest where I'd fallen on my purse, but the whole left side of my body was numb from shoulder to waist. Telling myself that the numbness was just a temporary reaction to the fall, I dressed and went to work. I would be fine. Without paying very much attention to it, I believed it would go away. Because I had always enjoyed good health, I felt immune from such problems. Pushing out of my mind any memory of the strange loss of sensation in my legs, I avoided the reality that there had been no bump, crack, or dip in the smooth pavement to have caused my fall. Since the numbness in my torso didn't impede my functioning, I ignored it and kept on going. I had things to do, obligations to meet, and a life to live.

My condition, however, did not go away; it got worse. In mid-December, I awoke one morning to find that my whole left leg, toes to groin, was totally numb. When I tried to walk, it was like dragging a log around, and when I put weight on my left foot, I couldn't feel the floor. Still, I got dressed and went to work; it never occurred to me to do otherwise. Slowly and laboriously, I dragged myself from the parking lot to my office. Once there, I really didn't have to move all that much. As a psychotherapist, I sat in sessions, getting up only to escort a client in or out of my office. So once there, I set to work.

By midmorning, however, I could no longer keep ignoring my situation and I mentioned what had happened to the nurse in my office. Only at her urging did I make an appointment with my family doctor, irritated that I had to change my schedule to accommodate his. The doctor ordered an MRI for my head and cervical spine, which was normal. Then I had an EMG (a test that measures conduction of impulses in the peripheral nerves) of my legs to see if that was the location of the problem. That too, came back normal. And so, with no clear clinical sign of disease, my doctor suggested that my symptoms might be transitory and that we take a wait-and-see approach. That fit my pattern of ignoring and denying just fine.

Over the next few weeks, my symptoms did subside a bit, just enough to give me hope. I continued to work full time, but that was about all I was able to handle. The tiredness that had been building all summer and autumn became my constant companion. After my fall, it had transformed into a type of fatigue I had never encountered before, a kind of mental and physical paralysis that overcame me whenever I overtaxed my limited energy. As he would do for the next year, my husband took over most of the household tasks, and I was even forced to stop attending my daughter's volleyball games. By the end of February, my right foot was also engulfed in a constant numbness and tingling that would, at various times, creep up that leg as well. With this new symptom added to my still-numb torso and lower left leg, there was little I could do physically.

As I look back on that time, I realize that, as my disease numbed me physically, I was also numbing myself mentally and emotionally in order to keep going. I never missed a day of work, which—with my sons away at school most of the year, my daughter in high school, and my husband taking charge of the household—is where I thought my primary responsibility now lay. Though limited, I kept up with my family as best I could. I was an automaton, damaged and defective, who mindlessly kept going on the life path that seemed to me necessary and essential.

As February turned to March and then April, more symptoms appeared, though I tried to ignore them. My left cheek would become tight and painful; I'd have tingling in my hands, and, at odd hours, an excruciating headache on the left side of my skull. And there was still the relentless fatigue that, when it washed over me, rendered me unable to think and filled me with such lethargy that I could barely move—and didn't want to, even if I could. But despite my tiredness, at night my legs were so painful that I couldn't sleep. By then, I was so emotionally drained that I found myself crying much of the time. One morning, I woke up with both arms numb. I panicked—it was bad enough that I could barely walk, but what would I do without the use of my arms?

Fear of the Unknown

MS is a terrorizing disease: it can attack at any time, anywhere in your body, with symptoms lasting a moment, an hour, a day, or forever. For a person with MS, odd sensations, pains, weaknesses, and changes in vision are daily occurrences. Because any symptom can strike at any moment, leaving one helpless and ashamed, one lives in constant fear. Dreading what will be lost next, and feeling powerless to do anything about it, wears on the spirit. So even though my new symptoms turned out to be transitory, coming and going at their whim, they took a terrible toll.

By May, my condition had deteriorated even more. I could barely walk, and climbing stairs was a nightmare. I couldn't tell when my left foot had landed, so it was a very slow process to trudge up or down, always leading with my right leg. I had no life left in me; all my energy had been drained. I returned to the doctor, who sent me back to the neurosurgeon for more MRIs. This time they took an image of the whole spine with an enhancing dye, which showed abnormalities, some white spots along the spinal cord and a bulging disk. The main diagnosis became that bulging disk, at least according to the radiologists.

The neurosurgeon, however, was not satisfied with the bulging disk explanation and ordered a spinal tap. The result came back with Ig bands, which are specific immune cells found in the spinal fluid. My ignorance protected me at the time because I didn't realize what those bands indicated—that my own immune cells were responsible for my symptoms. They were attacking the myelin sheath that acts as an insulator around the nerves, thus causing disruption in the nerve impulses. The neurosurgeon was very hesitant and ambiguous when he suggested that I might have MS. Of course, admittedly I was crying, and who wanted to deal with that? He ended our conversation with the recommendation that I seek a second opinion. And because he hedged, I maintained my ignorance, not knowing or wanting to know anything about MS. My denial that I might have the disease held fast.

Nevertheless, in his clumsy way he did me a favor by galvanizing me to finally take action. Soon, the Mayo Clinic confirmed his tentative diagnosis: lesions seen as white spots on the spinal cord, a definitive MS sign of scarring or sclerosis, were identified on my thoracic spine. Normally, the diagnosis of MS can take up to three years and visits to as many as eight doctors, so, although I certainly wouldn't have said so at the time, I was lucky to have my diagnosis within ten months of my first major attack. The sooner intervention begins, including the diet/nutritional treatment, the better the prognosis.

Betrayal

When I held my private pity parties, I felt angry and betrayed by my body and I despaired for the future. Nothing worked right, especially my legs. I obsessed about my MS, entertaining visions of life in a wheelchair, dependent on others. I felt guilty because I knew my wonderful husband would never abandon me, which meant his life, too, would forever be under the cloud of my disease. He would spend the rest of his years taking care of me. We tried to be both brave and realistic by discussing how we could modify the house to accommodate a wheelchair. And we also felt an urgency to take a few vacations before I got any worse, because I was losing ground quickly.

Along with all my obsessing came a brutal honesty. I recalled all the warning signs I'd had over the previous year—my never-ending fatigue, always feeling cold, never feeling "right." In truth, however, the biggest betrayal of all was my own for not honoring and taking care of my body. My body made a valiant attempt to fight off the disease, but I had given it no help. In fact, I had barely acknowledged it.

In a sense, I had moved out of my body years before, living from my shoulders up, acknowledging only my mind and will. If I willed myself to do something, I expected that I could no matter how my body felt or how taxing the task. I ate carelessly. We were a busy American family on the go, so we often grabbed something at a fast-food restaurant or at the concession stand when attending one of the children's events. Over the years I had gained weight, just a couple of pounds a year, but it added up. I rarely exercised; I didn't have time. I went to bed too late and got up too early. There was so much to do.

Even when I had my first attack, I never thought to cut back and give my body some loving care. I just expected to get back my health, as if it were my due. After all, I had never really been sick before. Now I realized for the first time how spoiled I had been by my good health. With this new insight, I recalled that about seven years earlier my left leg was tight and had pained me for several weeks. Back then, I was working only part-time, teaching a few days at a local college, and my activities were not so frenetic. I napped quite a bit, my problem went away, and I forgot about it. I also recalled a couple of years earlier when I had consulted an orthopedic physician about the pains in my legs. He told me that my description of the pain path made no sense and dismissed it. I should have followed up on that. Honesty compelled me to acknowledge a several-month struggle with incontinence a year or so earlier, which I had also done my best to ignore. It was humiliating and I never mentioned it to anyone. If only I had listened to my body in those years before my attack. These thoughts haunted me.

In retrospect, it is strange how we hold ourselves responsible for our diseases. In truth, I probably had the template for MS all along—the genetics, the original viral infections, the tendency to allergies and sensitivities, the environmental factors—and who knows if I could ever have avoided the disease's manifesting at that time or at another time.

My MS continued its march that summer of 1997. I'll forever remember how totally defeated I felt when I took a walk, holding on to my husband and moving at a snail's pace. Still, I couldn't make it any farther than three houses down the sidewalk before my legs and my energy gave out. I was also sleeping my life away. It seemed that I was able to function for no more than four to five hours before I had to rest. If I didn't, I was useless, and worse, my symptoms would escalate.

I Strike Back

It is not in my nature to accept anything passively, and certainly not this slow inexorable deterioration of my functioning. For ten months starting the night before Halloween 1996, I had struggled with a nameless tormentor, alternately denying, fearing, holding on to the smallest hope whenever I experienced a diminishing of symptoms, and despairing of my helplessness. From that point of view, August 1997 was a positive turning point for me because I finally knew the name of my adversary/

disease. Once I had it, I followed the old cliché: "Know thine enemy." Fighting the MS and restoring my health became the central focus of my life. I cut back at work, and when that still proved to be too much, I took a leave of absence. Then, with my freed-up schedule, I hit the bookstores and library to read all I could about the disease.

The books written by members of the medical establishment were all pretty bleak, offering no promise of improvement. For the most part, they were filled with advice on how to medicate symptoms and handle disabilities. They tried to set out categories and prognosticate the factors determining the level of disability, but gave no sense that any treatment could really do anything about the disease's progression. My own risk factors, that I was older and hadn't had a remission, predicted a bleak future. And what I read about the new drugs, the ABCs, did not inspire me; at most they were reported to do no more than slow the disease's progress, and they were often accompanied by a variety of unpleasant side effects. In any case, none of the doctors I had seen had even mentioned them as a possible treatment for me.

Luckily, Judy Graham's *Multiple Sclerosis: A Self-Help Guide to Its Management*, published in 1989, was still in the bookstores. A British journalist with MS, Graham wrote about the diet that had allowed her—like many others who were following it—to stop the progression of the disease and restore most of her abilities. I grabbed on to this nugget of hope, not only consuming her book but also hunting down many of the references in her bibliography, which is how I found *The Multiple Sclerosis Diet Book*, by Dr. Roy Swank and Barbara Brewer Dugan, another invaluable resource. Both books presented the idea that MS could be slowed, stopped, and sometimes reversed through diet and nutritional modification. After reading them, I knew with certainty that the nutritional approach was for me and that I would get better. In late August 1997, I began to follow their prescriptions for rest, exercise, and, most important, dietary changes.

Again, the Swank diet recommends a very low consumption of saturated fats, coupled with a high consumption of oils and an emphasis on eating fruits and vegetables. Fortunately, as it turned out, I chose to cut out dairy altogether even though Swank suggested eating only low-fat dairy. Swank's plan does not include the component of food sensitivity and the need to eliminate trigger foods. Dairy, as I learned later, is one such food for me, so cutting it out at this point was beneficial, though almost accidental on my part.

I began to swim every morning and hobbled to yoga. It was a struggle, but I was determined, and my teacher, who had found yoga crucial to her own recovery from a car accident, was both encouraging and helpful. I napped in the afternoon, not only because Swank suggested it in his book but also because, realistically, I needed the extra sleep in order to function. My MS stopped its downward progression. The numbness in my torso and then my leg diminished after about three to four months. Although transitory symptoms still appeared on occasion, they did so with less frequency, and there were no new enduring symptoms that, in MS language, would constitute a major attack or an exacerbation. The general trend was up.

As I continued to improve and to develop a greater sensitivity to my body, I began to believe that I could actually control the disease. In a very real way, my MS and my body became both my teachers and my taskmasters. I had to plan what I could do based not only on how much energy I had available but also on whether or not the activity was important enough to warrant the expenditure of what limited energy I had. With my physical activities limited to what I could realistically accomplish, I had no real choice but to live fully in my body. That meant listening to it and becoming sensitive to the ebb and flow of energy and feelings. If I pushed too much, I would be stopped by that paralyzing fatigue; if I overexerted, my symptoms would flare up.

Knowing that my disease would become my identity in many people's minds—"You know Ann Sawyer, the one who has MS"—I shared my diagnosis only with my family and close friends. Still, I felt shame at even having MS, at being flawed and disabled. Logic tells me that I shouldn't have felt that way, but I did. So the first real milestone in my recovery came when I could walk without a perceptible limp, which fortunately happened quite soon, within about three months for short distances only. It was important to me that my disease be hidden from public view. Although I couldn't at first maintain a smooth gait over any distance, I found that there was very little walking expected in modern life. Gallantly, my husband dropped me off at the door wherever we went, and picked me up when the event or visit was over. At most, I was required to walk no more than a couple of hundred feet. My pride was saved.

I'd still have hit-and-run attacks, as I called that array of symptoms that would torment me at odd times. But since none of these was new, and none appeared to be permanent, I was hopeful that I might be safe from another major attack.

My improvement continued in small increments. With the return of each ability, I celebrated. Funny little things that I'd never even thought about before, like being able to alternate feet when going up and down the stairs, were now precious skills. By the spring of 1998 I could walk a mile, albeit not at the fastest pace and with some increasing numbness over the distance; nonetheless, I was very pleased.

Much improved, I returned to work. Within weeks, however, my marked limp and other symptoms began to return. This put me in the terrible position of having to choose between my health and everything I believed about what I should be and what value I had to society.

"Just get a scooter," a longtime wheelchair-bound person with MS told me. But I'd seen what life was like for this person. As a medical doctor and researcher, he was able to continue working mainly because he didn't seem to have the cognitive or fatigue problems so often associated with MS. Still, his life was extremely limited, and I felt for his wife, who fought bitterness and depression. I didn't want that same fate for either myself or my husband.

My employer had been kind, but there was a limit to how long I could ask him to hold my job. As a psychotherapist, I was constantly trying to teach my clients to love and value themselves for who they were and not for what job they had or how they looked. At that point, I needed to take my own advice. I made the decision to quit work. It was hard to give up so much of what had been my identity, hard to place myself in the category of people with debilitating health problems. There was, however, really no choice; I needed the time for myself and my pursuit of health.

It didn't take long after I returned to my full program of diet, exercise, rest, and low stress that I was once again on the upswing. I had never abandoned the diet, but at that point in my recovery, the other components were equally important. After about a year and a half of slow improvement, however, I reached a plateau. It wasn't a bad place to be—the only symptoms left were a faint tightness in my left torso and a numb/tingling sensation in my lower left leg and both feet. The latter is much like the sensation one has when a leg goes to sleep: first there is the deadness, and then a tingling in decreasing intensity until normal feeling is restored. If I was tired or had a flare-up, the symptoms could get much worse, activating my left side headache, my cheek, and my hands. I was perhaps two-thirds of the way back to normalcy, with the numb/tingling sensation faint enough that it didn't interfere too much with my walking. To my chagrin, however, the fatigue continued to plague me.

Believing that I could do better if I only had the right key, I began to seek more information. Although in my reading I had seen some references to the association between food allergies or sensitivities and MS, I had been unable to find any substantive information on the subject. Knowing this, my more technologically advanced husband hit the Internet. By chance, among the 5,000 or so sites for MS listed on the Web at that time, he found a paper by Ashton Embry titled "Multiple Sclerosis: Probable Cause and Best Bet Treatment." Embry, a research scientist by profession, had been frustrated by the lack of good medical knowledge of and treatment for MS when his son was diagnosed. Having come upon Roger MacDougall's and other writings about the diet/nutritional approach, he began to gather current and historical research on the treatment, making it available to the lay public and lobbying the medical establishment to seriously consider its validity. The paper my husband found not only laid out the theory behind the diet/nutritional treatment but also gave a complete blueprint for recovery.

Hungry for all the knowledge and insights I could possibly find, I read and reread every word, and followed up by reading some of the references. What Embry had to say made complete sense to me intellectually and conformed to my own experience of the disease. His nutritional treatment incorporated much of the work done by others before him, including Roger MacDougall's discovery that wheat was a trigger and Swank's theories about fat. Embry took the diet/nutritional treatment to a much more sophisticated level by determining that sensitivities to foods other than gluten could be responsible for triggering symptoms as well as by focusing on other body systems compromised in MS and ways to facilitate healing them as well.

I took the ELISA test, which measured my immune response to 190 foods. Not surprisingly, the results were consistent with Embry's theory: I registered sensitive to many foods. I immediately eliminated these foods from my diet and my improvement curve again sharpened.

As I read what Embry had to say about food sensitivities, an experience from the year before came to mind. At the time I had been following Swank's low-fat approach, so I had ordered what I thought was a safe dinner of shrimp marinated in egg white. As I lay in bed several hours later, however, my legs hurt so much that I took the only prescription medication I had been prescribed for managing my MS. It was a strong painkiller, but even so, it did not alleviate the pain. Finally, that experience and others like it began to make sense. As it turns out, egg whites are one of the foods to which I'm most sensitive.

Food—the answer seemed almost too easy to be true. But when I thought about it, we eat different foods every day; some days we may have nothing that triggers MS, while on others we may eat many offending foods. So, depending on how far the disease has progressed, on the days when we consume no food triggers, we may have no symptoms or our symptoms could remain at low ebb. Then, on a day when we eat several foods to which we are sensitive, our MS symptoms abound. Simple? Yes, but that is essentially how I have found it to work.

Continuing on the diet, I came to know my body so well that patterns began to emerge. Instead of an unknown specter that attacked me for no reason, my MS, I now saw, was actually operating according to the laws of cause and effect. If I eat that, I will have symptoms; if I eat only these foods, my symptoms will diminish. I regained some of my natural buoyancy because I no longer feared the disease. Once again, I had some power over my life and hope for a better future.

With joy, I found that after about six months of following the advice in Embry's article, I could take the stairs at a fast clip and walk long distances. But I wanted more. Further healing depended on my becoming even more finely tuned to my disease, my body, and the interaction between the two. Again, MS is a disease that manifests itself uniquely in each individual, with a wide array of possible symptoms that also vary in duration and intensity. Even with relation to its clinical signs, MS is a mystery. There is no correlation either between the number of lesions and the degree of disability or between the location of the lesions and the type or location of symptoms. MS follows no neat path or rules.

By listening to and watching my disease and my body's reactions, I continued my self-education. When my symptoms flared up, I could usually figure out why and then correct my diet. Sometimes I had to test and verify my assumption, as one might do in a laboratory. In a way, I became my own lab rat.

At that point, it wasn't just food that affected my MS. Colds, the flu, fatigue, stress—anything that caused my immune system to react, including my menses—would trigger an increase in symptoms. It's easy to say don't get sick, but much harder to do. In addition, I was still struggling with extreme fatigue on a daily basis. The cruelest twist was my discovery that joy and elation are also stressors. At my daughter's high school graduation, I was so proud and happy, my leg went numb and I had to hold on to my husband for support. It seemed that my teachers—the MS and my body—were insisting that I learn serenity.

As my healing progressed, I found that my fatigue lessened and stress and sickness no longer triggered an increase in symptoms. I can only attribute this continued improvement to time and patience in letting my body heal and strengthen against the disease. There is a lot yet to be understood about this disease and all its effects on the body, but I don't need to understand exactly why something works in order to appreciate my increased energy and hardiness.

By midsummer of 2000, I was feeling fine. More abilities returned: I could skip, jump up and down, and even stand on one leg long enough to put on panty hose. I now take secret glee in wearing high heels—just because I can.

In the fall of 2000, with only some fuzziness remaining in my feet, I hiked about two-thirds of the way down the Grand Canyon, to Plateau Point and back, in one day. It is a trek of twelve miles, covering an elevation change of three thousand feet. And, without wanting to embarrass my friend Nora, I must say that I had to slow down for her sake when she was finding it difficult to go the last mile or so.

8

Judi's Story

When I was sixteen years old, I went on a trip with my boarding school to the Mount Snow ski resort in Vermont. Little did I know what this outing would bring. The day before, I had gone hiking with a friend up the shoulder of a Berkshire mountain behind our school. Although early snowmelt had partially cleared the trails, the higher we went, the more snow we encountered. By midday, I was up to my thighs in cold white drifts, soaked through, and ready to give up. My male friend persevered, and I was not about to be left behind. I was exhausted but exuberant on our return down the mountain, and slept soundly that night to get up at dawn for the promised ski trip.

I was dressed for the occasion although I had never really skied before. My mom had taken me to Macy's department store in New York City over Christmas vacation to get appropriate attire off the sale rack we found, and I was thrilled by my own sporty costume. When my school group arrived at our destination, we all got outfitted with the very long skis and heavy boots available in those days. Then it was off to the "bunny" slope to learn how to stand up without falling over, and perform the famous wedge-shaped snowplow maneuver to carefully execute basic turns across the slopes and how to come to a complete stop.

I was so happy with my progress at the lunch break that I was ready to try a real run down the mountain by myself. I hadn't counted on peer pressure. "Come with us," a bunch of guys shouted over a final cup of hot chocolate. "We'll get you on and off the chairlift safely. Come *on*!" So up we went to dizzying heights and saw the panorama of skiers both graceful ("not me," I thought) and those who were falling down all over the wide expanse of the trail below us. True to their word, the guys helped me off the lift, and then said, "Bye, have fun," and left me at the top of a very steep trail. This wasn't the bunny slope. It didn't look like fun to me at all.

Petrified, I scooted my way down very slowly, snowplowing from side to side directly parallel to the incline and sidestepping inch by inch down the slope. I finally gave up altogether, removed the skis with trembling fingers, and trudged down in my concrete boots to hand the whole mess in at the rental counter. I decided that mastering speed on thin wooden slats was not my thing. For the rest of the afternoon, I swam in the heated outdoor pool. I gazed up at my tall white nemesis beyond the fence, covered with people who actually liked this sport, and sighed deliciously as I sank underwater and swam to the other end of the pool.

When it was time to go, I could hardly get my body up the ladder. I tried to lift myself out several times before I crumpled into a heap at the pool's edge. "I must be really tired from yesterday," I thought. I waited a bit before I could finally get out and hurry off into a very cold shower. What followed became a legendary story from my childhood. I barely made it off the bus back to school, staggered inside for dinner, and fell asleep right into my mashed potatoes. The next day, I didn't get out of bed or go to classes. Everyone thought I was just faking it and was probably too sore to get up.

Not generally given to hypochondria, I managed to live down that story and returned to my life as vigorously as ever. Now my MS specialist doctor and I can look back and see the whole incident as the beginning signs of MS. Before there were MRIs and spinal taps to confirm the diagnosis, putting people into hot tubs was a good way to see the results of a body's inability to tolerate heat, which is often an MS indicator. If they couldn't get out, they probably had MS. Long before I was diagnosed with the disease at age thirty-five, the origin of these symptoms was invisibly working away inside my central nervous system getting ready to bloom again when the circumstances were right. The activities of so much unaccustomed exercise, followed by the heated swimming pool, proved to be the perfect stresses for my body to give me a warning sign that I totally ignored in my immortal youth.

The Birth of MS

My second daughter's birth was traumatic. I had an abrupted placenta, meaning that the placental sac had separated from the uterine wall during the forty-five-minute precipitous labor, which deprived her of oxygen at some point in delivery. By the next day, she went into severe respiratory distress and was taken by ambulance to the closest neonatal ICU, an hour away from home. After that day, I was on my feet for a whole week, hovering over her in the hospital and again when at last she came home. When it was clear that she had experienced seizures within hours of birth, creating unknown amounts of brain damage, I dealt with my fear, rage, and finally relief that she was going to live as best I could.

When she first came back with us to our house, I tried to return to the way-it-would-have-been. I stayed in bed as if she had just been born. I rested in the postbirth bliss that I remembered after her older sister's birth. But that was not the reality this time around. Not only had the bliss been shattered by my own feelings, but I had an active, jealous four-and-a-half-year-old on my hands.

My first daughter's worst fears must have been confirmed. The baby comes, almost dies, and her parents are totally focused on this new being. She could taste the fear in the air all around her previously safe life. When asked what it was like to have been at the home birth of her little sister, she replied thoughtfully, "Well, it was kind of like falling off a jungle gym." She hit upon an accurate analogy.

I wanted to give as much as I could to her transition to sisterhood. I could not make believe that this shock wave didn't happen to our family. My husband and I had been incredibly close, but he had to go back to work. He was the one to field the outpouring of well-intentioned questions about our new daughter's health, day after day. We were both exhausted and determined to get our lives back to normal.

Unraveling

We thought we had achieved that goal. But five months later, I felt my right leg start to go a little numb. I was tired, no doubt about it. I had a tunnel vision experience for a day or so. I thought it must have been "new-mother fatigue" when it disappeared. Maybe the numbness in my leg was because I hurt my lower back while mucking out the horse stalls with my baby in her backpack carrier? But the numbness spread farther over the first leg and then the other leg began to numb out, too. I made an appointment with my chiropractor.

My mother had been diagnosed with multiple sclerosis in her late fifties. It was only a little question in the far corner of my mind, but I needed to ask it. I couldn't believe that I might have her disease.

My chiropractor looked me over, agreed that this was most likely stress induced, and said cheerily, "No, it isn't MS." I went to bed very relieved. But the numbness steadily got worse. Finally, I could feel nothing from my waist down. When I lay on the bed with my eyes closed, my sense of feeling stopped at my belly button. My chiropractor immediately referred me to a neurologist, the same one my mother used. He asked a lot of questions, gave me a basic neurological exam, and said, "I think you have MS." He couldn't be sure without blood tests and spinal taps but he felt that it was.

I was speechless. I didn't understand all of the ramifications of the diagnosis at that time. The doctor said that sometimes these symptoms are the result of a virus that women can contract after giving birth. I clung to that for a while. I clung to anything that could take this illness away. Maybe all the blood work would come back with normal results. Did I really have to have a spinal tap? He also suggested I have an MRI. That might help him to confirm the diagnosis even though, sometimes, the sclerosis or plaque on the sheathing of the central nervous system doesn't show up. It certainly wouldn't help him to heal me. Western medicine didn't offer much at that time, except drugs to minimize the effect of the numbing.

It was in December, a couple of weeks before Christmas. I got all the blood work done, and the spinal tap, too. Although inconclusive, the results of the tests supported my doctor's original diagnosis; my body appeared to be fighting MS.

Merry Christmas

The holiday season was grim that year. The original onset of symptoms made physical the worst fear I have ever known. The numbness kept creeping deeper and deeper into me, until my legs were like two wooden logs connected for some reason to the rest of my body. I could barely stumble up the stairs. I didn't dare carry the baby anywhere for fear of falling with her. I was so exhausted, that I went to bed whenever I could. I never woke up refreshed. There was a hole in me where my life was running out, and deadness was the only sign that there had ever been life at all.

Everyone around us was shocked, too. I appreciated people's honest responses. I preferred, "I don't know what to say, first the baby, now this—I can't believe it," to statements like, "It will be all right soon, don't worry." Everybody suggested a thousand things to do as a way of coping with the fear.

The month following the onset of my symptoms was filled with unknown possible horrors. Would I become so bad that I could no longer make it upstairs to our bedroom? Should I move downstairs? Would I ever be able to drive again? Living in the country, this was a big one. At that time, I couldn't even feel the pedals of the car. Family and friends helped enormously with running the house and looking after the children. But they had their own busy lives. What kind of permanent help would I need? It was so hard to think that I couldn't mother my own children.

The doctors had no answers either. MS is such an unpredictable illness. Its course could be slow and subtle or swift and mercilessly crippling. Probably this initial attack would subside somewhat, but when? In what condition would it leave me? Remissions are possible, but every renewed attack would leave increased damage to my nerves. How often would the attacks come? Would I become a complete cripple, bound to a wheelchair? Thoughts like these tormented me while I tried to carry on my everyday life, swimming uphill against a deep well of exhaustion.

Fear pulsated like an evil being throughout the household. Sometime in February, the worst of the numbness began to remit. My symptoms receded gradually. I used to be a dancer and working with my body to make it stronger and more flexible was something I had always taken for granted. No more.

Dancing with MS

Denial of an acute or chronic disease and its effects is a common reaction. Like most of us with MS, I had continued my busy life "as usual" despite remonstrance from family and friends. I justified my insistence to be "normal" by claiming it as a positive attitude. I didn't want to acknowledge the toll that it took upon my beleaguered system. In fact, I was perpetuating all the stressful systems from the past and compiling that stress by pushing a body that had already reached its limits months ago. Routines, however detrimental, are familiar, and I was loath to give a single one of mine away.

Unlike Ann, I avoided too much research about MS because I was so frightened by the dire predictions that were then available to me. Instead, I went about exploring as many "alternative" healing practices as I could. One of the first alternative healing experiences I pursued was the hands-on healing services of a friend and colleague, Barbara Brennan. Barbara gave me hope. After our sessions, I could feel my physical symptoms shifting, although not as dramatically as I wanted. In those early years, I had on healing blinders. I wanted a complete cure for my suffering, and nothing less than a miracle would do. Healing as a process was not acceptable to me.

Somewhere in the world, at this very moment, someone has had a complete remission from this incurable disease. I have met people who have told me their miracle story of complete remission from cancer, MS, and other illnesses. But that may or may not become my story. How do you hold on to believing in the possibility of a cure while fully embracing the long road to step-by-step healing and loving the miserable effects of this disease? The most important gift I received from Barbara was when she said: "Judi, this is the rest of your life in terms of your body. You must slow down. You must rest, sleep, for several hours every single day. How you heal yourself now, after this first attack, is for the remainder of your physical existence."

"Sleep for three hours every day? Impossible! My children, my psychotherapy practice, my country life with two horses, three gardens, my cats, my dog, my presidency of the school board, the rest of my life? Go away from what I know is me, to be alone and sleep with me, who is sick, maybe forever?" It seemed an insurmountable task to even contemplate.

As I look back on it, this was perhaps the most poignant moment since hearing my diagnosis. In the process of grappling with the information that you now have a debilitating illness for the rest of your life, at some point you must give up the life that *was*, in the uncompromising necessity to make room for the life that is.

Facing that choiceless choice was the difference between a life of rejecting or embracing the path that lay before me. I stepped off the clearly defined road maps of my previous expectations into the uncharted territory of my inner self. I had only viewed my life before through the lens of a healthy body.

In the end, because I knew that it was the prudent thing to do, I hired a lovely young woman to help me five days a week. It took several months of interviews and false starts before the right person appeared. I listened to myself explain to different women why I needed their help with my children. Having the illness as an incontrovertible fact gave me permission to ask for that help. It was an uncomfortable stance at first. But gradually I realized how unused I was to saying, "No, I can't do that anymore." I had always looked for ways to be an indispensable doer.

Resigning from my position on the school board was actually a relief by the time I divested myself of my responsibilities there. My therapy practice was not very large at the time, and keeping it that way was simple. Once the right mother's helper had settled in, and I realized how much loving, enthusiastic energy she had to give to my children, I adapted to the new routine.

For the first few months, I walked into my office, separated from the noises of my family, as if I were to face a firing squad. I didn't want to feel the level of exhaustion that kept shooting me down, day after day. I devised little rituals to ease the transition from "I must keep going" to "I must rest and heal."

Many Modalities of Healing

For the next many years, I worked with a variety of alternative modalities, or holistic healings, in addition to hands-on healing. The words *health* and *whole* come from the same Old English root; holistic, or whole, therapies are healing therapies. Some basic descriptions of all these alternative therapies that I explored are listed in Appendix C.

I also swallowed many supplements, in tincture, powder, and capsule form. Some are still recommended as good support for people with MS today (these are listed in Appendix A), and others were particular to my specific metabolic needs. All of the practitioners were highly qualified in their respective field, and each exploration gave birth to new understandings of the mystery we call a human being. None of them brought me a "cure" for MS or even a reduction or remission of symptoms.

One method I called upon in the very beginning and still use daily was simply to pray and meditate. That is not as easy as it sounds. Back then I had to struggle with what I could honestly pray for. I wasn't in the mood to dabble. I now have a client who calls New Age "Newage," to rhyme with "sewage." I knew what she meant. I didn't want to "be responsible as a co-creator" of this illness as much of my New Age training dictated. I didn't have the energy for anything but the truth. I found myself trying to protect my idea of God, Spirit, or Consciousness from my anger.

Anger is another common reaction after the denial begins to fade. It was hard to admit that I only wanted to pray for immediate release from this form of suffering. "I want to go back to the way I was living before. I don't want to learn anything from my present afflictions, I only want out! Someone has to take the blame for this and it isn't me." I looked for someone or something to blame. When I allowed myself to have a conscious dialogue in my own head, I could hear the underlying pain and confusion in the childish assumption that someone was to blame. I was trapped as long as I remained bound by this belief in guilt. As a victim, I was powerless to pray for anything that could take off my blindfold and face the enemy of my struggles. Taking responsibility for creating events in my life could so easily be misused. It was a small step off that fine line of truth into, "If I'm ill, I created it. Illness is bad. I must be bad to have created my illness," and, conversely, "If I'm good, then it will go away."

When the time is ripe for self-investigation, being responsible *to* your illness, to want to know *why* from the depths of your being, brings a wealth of discovery that makes the inner journey an enriching one. If I am co-creator of my illness, albeit on deeply unconscious levels, then I am also co-creator of my healing. That was the beginning of a new outpouring of self-love that emerged from holding my disease in the light of truth and heightened awareness. Eventually, I found heartfelt prayers appropriate for each day. I poured out my sorrows, my confusions, my daily wrestling matches with life, which were highlighted by the fatigue that dogged me. After yelling or crying or quietly entreating for help in finding clarity and courage, I surrendered in relief to the sleep that followed.

Questions I have asked myself along the way are: Would I really be much happier if I could take a long walk in the woods right now? If I could help with the dishes after dinner at a friend's house, does that mean the friend would love me more? If I could go to the store for groceries, stand in a long line to pay, and then run home to do a load of laundry, would that make me a better person? If I am honest, the answer is no; I cannot know these things to be true. I cannot believe that fulfilling these desires would bring me peace. If I insist they would, I create my own suffering. Besides my alone time used in prayer, I also used many forms of visualizations and meditations. I used techniques of looking at my body as healthy. At night, I sometimes had joyful dreams of walking barefoot in the mud or on a grassy lawn, and would realize in the morning that my feet still knew how to have full sensory feedback somewhere inside of my brain. I would use these remembered sensations to infuse my visualizations with some eros for health.

Building Faith

It was now clear I did indeed have the kind of MS that was going to take me on a steady slide downhill, without severe relapses, but with no clear remissions, either. My alternative therapies were all good for me (and I think actually did slow down my decline), but still my symptoms increased. In the fall of 1999, I finally decided to try one of the ABC medications touted to slow the progression of MS. Some relapsing-remitting MS clients who had just been diagnosed were on Avonex, and although they suffered flu-like symptoms the one day a week they gave themselves an intramuscular injection, their MS progress might indeed have been slowed down. I recommended Avonex to any newly diagnosed client who called me for advice. Someone else who was a student in my movement classes with a long-term case similar to mine felt dreadfully ill after a month on Avonex and switched to Copaxone, which requires an everyday subcutaneous injection. No one I knew was on Betaseron.

Five years earlier, I had an appointment with Dr. Murray Bornstein, the "father of Copaxone" as he was called in a pamphlet. At that time he gave me the most thorough exam I had ever had from a neurologist. He was past the age of needing fame and glory from his thirty-plus years of research with MS. He said, "I have a recent videotape in my closet of an old MS client tap-dancing. When she was on my drug in the experimental phase, she was in a wheelchair. Do I know if it was my drug that got her out of it? I cannot know. Don't take my drug or any drug that is out there right now. None of them are clearly helping to do anything except make someone's career. We just don't have enough information yet. We will understand autoimmune diseases so much better one day, with all the new technology at our disposal. Just go home, keep doing what you are doing, and remyelinate."

This was amazing to me. I had never heard such an optimistic and truthful physician before. I felt his support when he said to me to, "Stop saying relapse and remission. Just eliminate those ideas from your vocabulary and see what happens." For the first time with a neurologist, I felt that he really wanted me to get better by myself. It wasn't about him at all. I wanted to go home and do just what the doctor ordered. But for me, there were no permanent good results from all of the alternative methods I had under my belt. When I saw him back then, I was in much better shape than I was now, and Copaxone had not yet been stabilized for reliable manufacture. Now I was scared and thought, "What have I got to lose if I do try a drug?"

I debated a long while about this decision. I didn't like the idea of shooting myself with 10,000 times the amount of the protein interferon that my body naturally makes as an anti-inflammatory agent. I also heard that Avonex doesn't hold up well statistically for slowing down the progression of decline with my kind of secondary progressive MS.

Biting the Medical Bullet

I felt so poorly at the time that I finally resigned myself and asked my insurance company to look into their payment plan for me on Avonex. It offered terrible coverage. I switched insurance companies and was finally all lined up to get the drug delivered to my door that week, when a client of my husband's suggested I try a new drug, Prokarin (formerly known as Procarin). The information on this new drug was only available on the Internet, as the FDA did not yet approve it. I checked out the website. The woman who invented it, Elaine DeLack, suffered from MS herself before she rediscovered a theory and the resulting drug based on Dr. Bayard T. Horton and Dr. Hinton Jonez's forgotten research from the 1930s to the 1950s (see the bibliography). My reading of her proposed theory about the neurotransmitter histamine was the first time that some of my own burning questions were answered as to how and why MS worked in so many confusing ways.

I canceled my first Avonex delivery and instead got a prescription of Prokarin ordered for me by a doctor friend. She researched it and said it was very benign and could do no lasting harm to my body. Best of all, I would know inside of a week if it worked for me or not. It wasn't about the invisible effect of possibly slowing progression; it might actually help to relieve my current symptoms. I knew my local neurologist wouldn't want to help me try out an unproven drug unless I could show him it was effective first. Although it was perfectly legal to prescribe, as the ingredients were all separately approved by the FDA (essentially they are histamine and caffeine mixed in a cream that is absorbed transdermally or through the skin), the ingredients were not approved as a mix for MS. I found a local compounding pharmacist (they make individualized medications from the basic ingredients) and with skeptical optimism tried Prokarin. It was interesting to challenge the mind-set of despair that had become deeply ingrained once again.

Life with Prokarin 1/20/00

Prokarin initially made a huge difference for me, even though after a year and a half, it was clear that it had ceased helping me the way it has helped others. Shortly after beginning on Prokarin, I was sitting in my morning bath, when I wondered who could have opened the window in January. My toes were freezing cold. I looked down at them and realized for the first time in years that they were cold because they were sticking up out of the water. I could feel my toes once again! Then I had to deal with a rush of passionate desire that this should never end, ever again. Hope is heady stuff. I thought it through and saw that with or without symptoms, I am still the same being. I could just enjoy the ride however long it lasted.

I had several phone calls and e-mail exchanges with Elaine DeLack asking questions about her drug for some of my clients. She gathered that I had movement experience and surprised me by asking if I would make a videotape for her company about the importance of exercise and Prokarin. I accepted her proposal and made a video titled *Prokarin, Movement, and MS.* I wanted this tape to help people at all stages of disability, whether they were bedridden, in a wheelchair, or still ambulatory, as I am. I was content with the result, and people with MS have responded by saying it was fascinating work and encouraged them to start moving again. I am pleased to think so.

I continued physically waxing and waning even while taking Prokarin. Walking the beautiful landscape of my home was a great gift that temporarily returned. I was sorry that it ultimately wasn't the answer for me as it has been for Elaine DeLack and others. Here was another opportunity to keep my heart open in the midst of disappointment.

Taking the Hit

In spite of Prokarin, I continued to decline. The exhaustion I felt increased, the rebound effect after using up muscular strength slowed to nothing, and I was losing my trunk muscles so that even sitting up was too exhausting. Even a wheelchair would never have worked.

After I crawled up the stairs to my room on all fours, I spent most of my days lying around in bed for hours, punctuated on a good day by one grueling excursion to the grocery store, during which I would pray that I wouldn't meet anyone I knew so I wouldn't have to say, "Sorry, I'm too tired to say hello right now." I had to grip the handle of the shopping cart to make one circuit around the store, throwing things into the cart without looking at them. My husband was torn between thinking I was too ill even to drive the seven minutes into town, and understanding that I had to at least try to get out of the house while he was working. Knowing that I couldn't sit up long enough for a wheelchair to have helped me out, I found myself envying people who could use them. What little capacity I had to pretend that I had some kind of outer life was slipping away rapidly.

I had been having inflammatory pain in my right sacroiliac joint (in the lower back, above and beside the tailbone) more and more frequently. If I stood for more than thirty minutes at a time, or tried to sit up for the same length of time, my back screamed at me in pain. Finally, it became chronic pain. I had no abdominal muscular strength to pull up and out of my back anymore. Later, this inflammation traveled right up my spine and into my trigeminal nerve, creating awful headaches.

Even sitting down, I was resting directly on my bones with no padding from my flaccid muscles, which aggravated an already weakened sacral area. Lying around all day in bed created other problems for me. I couldn't rest directly on my back, but had to prop myself up on one side or the other. I couldn't hold a book to read like that for very long, so my husband bought me a radio to listen to in bed. Still, I felt exhausted all day long. With virtually no exercise, I became even weaker. I could hardly move my bowels at all.

My local neurologist had me take heavy-duty steroids for three days, but for me it was an awful experience. I felt like a pumped-up empty paper bag and could hardly recognize myself, as my own hostility spilled out to everyone around me. My husband finally said that as my main caretaker, he needed to have me see an MS specialist in Manhattan, no matter what. I was too weak and in despair to do anything but agree. I surely couldn't let myself get worse without trying everything, including allopathic medications, no matter what I thought of their poisonous nature.

This neurologist was thorough and assured me that he could stop the progress of my MS symptoms. He explained to me that, indeed, MS is not one illness, and that the different medications he would have me try would address either general inflammatory responses using a chemotherapy called Novantrone, a B-cell malfunction that could be treated with transfusions of gamma globulin, or a T-cell dysfunction, which was countered by using one of the CRAB drugs. In fact, I consecutively did all three (including small doses, or "pulses," of intravenous steroids, which seem to tighten up the blood-brain barrier). I began taking Copaxone, despite what Dr. Bornstein said to me years ago.

I do credit the combined drug protocols with stopping the progress of my disease. But I was still lying in bed most of the time, too weak to do more than one short outing each day. I was also taking 4AP, or aminopyridine, to decrease the amount of potassium which is used in alternation with sodium chloride (salt) by the neurons to produce neurological electricity. This gave me a little more muscular strength. My first physical therapist suggested I take a drug called ProVigil for greater energy. On a good day, these both helped me to get out of bed for an extra hour at a time. Not much had really changed; I still was prone to vicious headaches, was too weak to sit up, and still incapable of leading a real life. I was left wondering when Western medicine might find a way to eliminate this disease from my body.

Recovery Diet

I met Ann through an old friend of mine who knew we were both women with MS and had a similar outlook on life. I liked her immediately as we met over tea in my hometown. At that first meeting, Ann gave me a copy of her original book, which I read as soon as I got home, and that night went on the Recovery Diet. I didn't know at the time she thought me in pretty bad shape, though she was impressed by my determination and knowledge of my own body.

I was familiar with some of the rudiments of this diet years ago during my younger daughter's health crises of epilepsy. I ate no meat (saturated fats) and no milk products, as I was basically a vegetarian and took many good supplements. At various times, I also tried eliminating gluten, sugar, and caffeine. Back then, I had developed severe candidiasis and I definitely had developed leaky gut syndrome as a result. At the time I tried my limited version of the Recovery Diet eighteen years ago, I had two small children, one quite ill, my own mother was dying, and I was overstressed and still looking for an immediate, complete cure.

When I met Ann, I was eating a basically healthy diet anyway—no red meat; organic and whole foods whenever possible—but I had not recently tried eliminating dairy, eggs, legumes, or gluten all at the same time. After one week on this diet, I regained feeling in my toes even more completely than I did on Prokarin, which has changed my walking for the better. After about six weeks, I also gained incrementally in terms of endurance and muscular rebound. In just the first month, it was exciting to feel renewed sensation moving up my legs and into my sacrum.

I was even able to walk back down to the waterfall on my land, to carry firewood, to empty the ash bucket, to make a spaghetti sauce, and to stay up to greet my husband on his late return from a trip to Florida, all in one day, and still felt just fine. There is no doubt that on this diet, my good days are definitely better.

Also, I had been getting vicious trigeminal headaches on just the right side of my head (like horrible migraines, only induced by inflammation of the fifth cranial nerve, the one that causes "ice cream headaches"). This occurred whenever I sat up too much, drove too much, talked with friends too long, stayed up too late or had any dental work done. It was further limiting my life, to say the least. The last time I had my teeth cleaned, I took nothing to prevent such a headache. I was taking Neurontin, both as a prophylactic and also when a headache started. This time, and without any support from the drug, I never got even a hint of a headache—no ice pick stabbing me in the eye!

The diet has had a profound positive effect on all of my symptoms. My doctor told me that if he had another life to dedicate to MS research (he is working with stem cells right now), he would investigate the effects of food. He sent me home as Dr. Bornstein once did: "Go home and see what more results you gain from whatever it is you are doing—including this diet. I support you in this experiment."

I am finding that this is no experiment. It isn't just an interesting hypothesis, it actually works. I continue to gain new sensations, mobility, strength, and endurance every month. Family and acquaintances alike tell me how different I look—how well, how animated, how strong. One relative told me how he saw all the lines of pain erased from my face. Best of all, their lovely comments simply mirror how well I am feeling inside.

Let me be specific about my gains. After eleven months, I stopped using Copaxone with no negative effect. I now have a life. I can spend most of a day out and about. I can drive to the nearest small city a half hour away and shop for clothes. Then I can stop for groceries, go browse among the library aisles for books (although I don't have as much time to read anymore), go home, pay bills, give a session, take the dog for a walk on the uneven ground in the woods, make dinner and clean up after, and sit up to watch a DVD movie in the evening.

As I regain feeling all over my body, I am amazed at how I could have walked at all several years ago. My left foot could barely lift off the ground, I had no volitional movement of my toes on that side, and the slump in my lower back with gravity pulling down into my right SI joint made moving my legs an agony of pain. When we went to a friend's house for dinner, I lay on a couch both before and immediately after eating, sometimes not even making it through the meal before I had to recline. I couldn't hold anything in my left hand without dropping it. I could finger-peck to type an e-mail, and start to cook a dinner but not always finish it, and that was with buying a lot of premade food. I wasn't interested in much beyond my bedroom walls.

When my long-term prognosis looked dim, my big hope was to be able to go grocery shopping and maybe do the laundry in the same day. When my symptoms were stabilized with drugs, I could plan to go to my daughter's college graduation by doing absolutely nothing for an entire week before and after the event.

Today I spend forty-five minutes every day exercising and working out. I can now wiggle those same toes and point and flex my left foot with some effort but also with great pleasure. I can lie down on my back without pain to go to sleep once again. I can trot up and down the stairs many times a day to cook, and clean house, make beds, give sessions, run errands, and write for several hours at a time. Although I still have to pace myself, I can fly on airplanes, navigating smaller airports without a wheelchair. I can sit up during long car rides to visit my far-flung daughters, walk down to our waterfall, harvest my little garden—

in short, I am gaining more strength and facility to live a normal life every day.

Today, I am daydreaming about hiking a lot more in the Catskills with my husband (with and without our future grandchildren), expanding our gardens, riding horseback again on these trails, and—some summer very soon—I have always wanted to go sea kayaking along the North Atlantic coast.

9

No One-Size-Fits-All Solution: Darlene

Challenge

One of the greatest challenges to the treatment of MS, no matter what the discipline or approach, is that the disease does not respond uniformly to any one intervention. In the world of allopathic medicine, the whole goal is to find that one specific medication that works for one specific disease. The early pioneers of the MS Recovery Diet approach had to learn the lesson of multiplicity and complexity as the treatment evolved.

As we've already discussed, Roger MacDougall was one of the early pioneers in the diet/nutritional approach to multiple sclerosis, not only in discovering some important components of the treatment, but also in his determination to spread the word.

He was a celebrated playwright and screenwriter (*The Mouse That Roared*, *The Man in the White Suit*, and *A Touch of Larceny*) when his mysterious illness progressed to the point that he lost his eyesight and was bedridden, unable to do even the simplest task. But his mind was active and his spirit determined. Using a parallel to celiac disease, another disorder where the body attacks itself, he came up with the notion that gluten is the culprit in MS. That was the case for him as it is for many others. He also decided to greatly limit fat intake, which had been researched and advocated by Dr. Roy Swank since the early 1950s. Sugar, the culprit in diabetes, was also eliminated. MacDougall gradually recovered full functioning and went on to write about his recovery and advocate the diet treatment. MacDougall died in 1993 at the age of eighty-two, still symptom-free.

In his early writings, MacDougall presented the diet that worked for him as the treatment for everyone. Many people with MS followed it, only to be disappointed because they did not enjoy the same recovery he achieved.

Darlene, profiled by Ann below, is one of the people who followed MacDougall's regime, but she also made some discoveries on her own. Her story illustrates how each person with MS needs to explore and discover the unique aspects of the disease and his or her body to formulate the diet that will work best.

An Uncommon Journey

At the time of the interview, Darlene was an elegant seventy-two-year-old woman. Her straight, proud posture and lively step belied her age. In her patrician features, etched with echoes of a million smiles, her character was revealed. There was a bounce to her step and a liveliness of spirit that radiated all around her.

Nothing in her appearance gave a hint that she had recently battled cancer. Her complexion glowed, her eyes sparkled, and her step was firm. Up until her then-recent illness, she judged herself to be in excellent health and doing much better than could be expected for her age. She and her husband led a happy, busy life and did volunteer and church work. Darlene was the image of how any woman would wish to be at seventy-two.

The Depths of Multiple Sclerosis

In 1974, Darlene's whole being was ravaged by her rapidly progressing multiple sclerosis. The overwhelming, paralyzing fatigue had robbed her of all vitality. "I was tired, I didn't care about anything," Darlene recalled. Her arms and legs were lost in numbness, preventing her doing any activity. Even worse, she was often beset with intermittent spasms, in which her muscles would tremor, and cramps, in which her muscles would tighten in excruciating pain.

MS also affected her vision, making the world a blurry place, taking away any possibility of reading or doing handwork. Darlene's cognitive abilities, like thinking and reasoning, were lost in an MS fog.

She became increasingly emaciated because, after eating, she experienced punishing pain in her chest and around her heart. Darlene added that another reason she got so thin was that often she was just too tired to chew and swallow. Finally, Darlene experienced difficulty swallowing and breathing, the last-stage symptoms.

Her days were spent sleeping or just lying down because she had neither the ability nor the energy to do anything else. Her wheelchair was too large for her house, so to get around she had to have someone help her or she'd crawl.

Twenty-eight years later, as Darlene recalled that time in her life, tears filled her eyes. "Our two daughters, who were teenagers, and my husband took over all the housework and cooking," she said with pride. "I'd be set up in the kitchen so I could give them some direction, but they did it all." Smiling through her tears, she expressed her pride and gratitude for her family's love and support.

Sharing Hope

Several years earlier, Darlene had given me two priceless gifts; the first hope, and the other new keys to the diet that would hasten my recovery. Through an acquaintance, I heard about Darlene's remarkable recovery and asked if I could meet her. Even though such a meeting meant that Darlene had to revisit those dark years, she graciously consented.

We talked for three hours, sometimes with tears, but also with laughter, as she dredged through her past to help me. To this day, I have almost total recall of that conversation, having often drawn on it for guidance and inspiration.

At that time, having already discovered many of the diet's components, I was making good progress in reclaiming my abilities. To do this, I had taken a leap of faith in trusting the written work of people I had never met. In all the writings I'd found, nowhere was there the promise of full recovery. Yet here was Darlene, a real, live person, who not only experienced the disease in its extreme, but also beat it. Her complete recovery had held for twenty-two years. Just meeting her gave me a powerful dose of hope and belief in my own future.

When I met with Darlene to do this profile, I explained how much her taking the time to meet with me and share her experience three years before had meant. She gave me a knowing smile. "That's how I felt about Roger MacDougall," she said, "even though I never met him."

MS Marches

At first, Darlene dated the start of her progressive MS to 1970, but paused and added, "Thinking back, I had symptoms for years before that." Dizziness and losing her balance were the first symptoms to appear. Oddly, she recalls always falling to her right. Next, she was plagued with weak and trembling legs. They were so bad that whenever she had to stop at a traffic light, she had to put her standard transmission car into neutral. She couldn't trust that her leg would stay on the clutch, so in order to insure the car stayed put, both feet were needed to keep the brake depressed.

In reference to these bothersome symptoms, I asked, "What did you do about them?"

Darlene chortled, "I tried to ignore them, thinking that they would go away." She went on to describe how she could will herself through anything, adding with a wry grin, "I have a very strong will."

In 1970, MS ceased to be a minor irritation that she could work around or ignore. Instead, it began to seriously and adversely affect her life. At that time, Darlene worked in an office just five minutes from her house, so she could go home for lunch. When the MS began to surge, she went home to sleep instead. To walk, Darlene was forced to hang on to the walls or furniture. Even with that, all too often she fell into large wastebaskets, Darlene said, grimacing at the memory. Still, she maintained her denial that anything was wrong, even as she began to use the restroom for naps over her breaks.

Her boss finally took action: he called her husband who in turn sent her to the doctor, who put her in the hospital. "They used to hospitalize people a lot back then," she explained. Since MS is an elusive, shadowy disease when it comes to diagnosis, the discovery that she had pernicious anemia took the blame for all her troubles. Darlene was immediately treated for that much more straightforward and manageable disease and sent home. Despite clearing up her anemia, she continued to decline. Back she went to the hospital for tests, followed by a referral to a neurologist.

Darlene has never forgotten her first visit to the specialist. First of all, he spoke only to her husband, as if she weren't present, and then ignored anything she did say, including her warning that she reacted poorly to tranquilizers. Without giving them any information or diagnosis, he handed her a prescription and said, "Take this, it will help you walk." He gave her no indication of his diagnosis, not an uncommon practice at the time, the thinking being that knowledge of what was wrong would just upset patients and do them no good. She took the medication and immediately had an adverse reaction. He had prescribed a tranquilizer.

Darlene returned to her family doctor. Over the next few years, Darlene says she was a guinea pig for any medication thought to be even remotely helpful to MS. Nothing helped; in fact, she had bad side effects and reactions to most of the medications. She continued to worsen and lost more and more of her abilities and energies.

Finding the Healing Path

"I always knew that I would heal. The Good Lord was with me, but I realized I had to do some of the work myself," Darlene explained. She was determined that she would not spend her life disabled.

Since conventional medicine failed to help, Darlene and Jack decided to look elsewhere for a treatment. With Darlene's vision and ability to think and reason compromised, Jack took on the task of reading and researching the disease and possible treatments. The first breakthrough came when a friend sent an article about how vitamin C and calcium were helpful in battling MS. Darlene immediately started taking them, experimenting with dosages.

The big breakthrough came when Jack found an article by Roger MacDougall in a 1974 issue of *Prevention*. Not only did he describe what to do, but he also had a special formula of vitamins and minerals, which he sold and Darlene bought. He incorporated the components he felt to be most important into his vitamins: B vitamins along with C, E, calcium, and magnesium. Darlene shared this article, her touchstone for healing, with me.

With nothing else to turn to, Darlene and Jack gave the diet their whole attention, as it was their only hope. She strictly adhered to MacDougall's proscriptions of no gluten, low sugar, low animal fat, and high oils, and the vitamin/mineral supplements. Following the recommendation that she ingest only pure substances, they distilled their own water. With a chuckle, Darlene explained that the contraption looked just like a gin still from Prohibition.

Beyond the MacDougall diet, they continued to research and add anything that made sense. From early on, Darlene drank a lot of water, half with lemon juice added, in the belief that it was important to cleanse her system. She also drank raw vegetable and fruit juices, which she made with her juicer. The live enzymes, vitamins, and minerals from the juice are easily absorbed, aiding in digestion.

Reading labels became a major part of meal planning. Darlene was amazed at how many additives, plus sugars and starches, are in our foods. To avoid these substances, they ended up making their own salad dressing and cooking mostly from scratch. MacDougall's diet only limits dairy fat, not dairy itself, so Darlene made her own yogurt using dried powdered skim milk.

"I was so desperate I would try anything," Darlene said with a laugh. "You wouldn't believe the extent to which I went." She proceeded to describe how, after hearing that wheatgrass juice was very beneficial, Jack went out and mowed some grass, which they then juiced. She drank it—regular yard grass. "We didn't know that wheatgrass was something different."

When I asked how she handled going out to eat, Darlene answered, "Those first years, I didn't go out. Sometimes, I'd try to go to church, but after getting dressed, I'd be too tired to go." She went on to describe an incident, after she had recovered some, when she attended a shower for someone close to her. It took a lot to just get there. "It hit me that I didn't even trust to drink the water." That is how dedicated she was to recovery.

Careful as she was in following the diet, after six months Darlene was discouraged because she felt that she hadn't registered any progress. Then, while praying, she realized that the pain in her chest and around her heart after she ate was gone. That one bit of progress was enough. She redoubled her efforts.

Darlene explained that she always tried to "remember the depths from which she had climbed," rather than look at all she still couldn't do. "That helps," she said, "as well as being aware of the little things. Recovery from MS is all about almost imperceptible steps forward." After a while, more confident, she began to vary her foods a little. "I noticed that some things on MacDougall's list didn't bother me," Darlene said. "And some of the things he said were okay did bother me." She kept a food diary, being especially careful to track new foods, which she introduced at a rate of one a week. For her, reactions to foods came quickly in the form of indigestion or echoes of past symptoms.

Darlene's most dramatic negative reaction was to yeast. Eggs, raw pears, white potatoes, and cantaloupe were other problem foods. "Actually," she observed, "I found any white food troublesome." This fits in with current research and thinking that highly processed foods, which have a high glycemic index, are bad for health. And her discovery of her own unique pattern of sensitivity to foods fits in with the current nutritional treatment for MS presented in this book.

There were many ups and downs during those healing years (fortunately, more ups than downs). Darlene also held through long plateaus, like not being able to walk. It was a good two years before she could hobble around on her weak and trembling legs, but it still opened her world. She could now get around her house and take care of things.

The telltale sign for Darlene was her digestion. If that was functioning poorly, she knew that she had triggered her MS to be more active. So it follows that her focus was then on good digestion and elimination. She had a history of constipation, so she took coffee enemas, a known remedy to natural healing. She consciously avoided any toxins and worked to cleanse her system by drinking lots of water and occasionally doing some sort of fast.

Over those years, Darlene became exquisitely sensitive to and in tune with her body. She said she could taste the food before she put it in her mouth. Through this process she was able to fine-tune her diet to her unique physiology. Not only did she discover which foods were harmful to her, she also found out which foods were healing and gave her strength. "Everything came together," she explained. "I eliminated the foods that gave me symptoms and ate enough of the right foods to make my body strong. It all got balanced."

In minute steps, Darlene kept getting better. "After I could walk without help, and it was hardly good walking, it took another two to three years before I could do stairs," she told me. Fortunately, her cognitive skills and ability to think and remember were among the first things to clear up. Her vision was another symptom that improved early on. This allowed her to read labels and do her own research on MS and nutrition.

Through the healing years, mindful that the anemia could return, Darlene had her trusted family physician monitor her. A good and compassionate man, he was supportive of her diet and was impressed by her results. Upon his request, she wrote up her experience, giving the details of what she did. Her doctor passed the essay on to some of his other patients with MS. None of them followed through, with one person going so far as to say that it was "too much work." Darlene noted that the same holds true now. She shook her head over all the unnecessary pain and suffering because of people's ignorance and unwillingness to take charge of their MS.

A Miracle

I asked Darlene how she knew she would beat MS. "I had healed before," she replied simply.

In 1963, Darlene had experienced another severe health crisis. She'd had rheumatic fever, with a white blood count no one could control. It left her weakened, with a heart murmur, and unable to walk without getting out of breath. Along with this she developed painful arthritis, so pervasive that most of her joints were swollen and painful. She was so sick that she had to do the unthinkable. It broke her heart to send their two young daughters to stay with grandparents, but she was unable to care for them. Darlene fully expected to die, even collecting some mementos to hand down to her daughters.

At that time, there was a faith healer in the news whose wife's cancerous tumor had disappeared miraculously. Apparently, the woman prayed and focused her mind on the tumor shrinking. Jack and Darlene were convinced that she, too, could be healed by faith. They directed all their prayers and energy to that end, even attending some of the revival services. Soon after, Darlene did experience an instantaneous healing. "Even my heart murmur is gone," she said, her voice still full of amazement and gratitude. Holding out her long, tapered fingers, she showed me that her joints had obviously returned to their normal size.

"After that, I just knew I could heal from the MS. But when the MS didn't clear up, it became clear to me that I had to do some of the work myself." She went on: "If it had been God's plan that I have MS and be in a wheelchair, I would have accepted it, but not without doing everything in my power to heal." She talked about the balance between acceptance of the disease and the determination to fight it with all she had. This attitude saved her from feeling sorry for herself and giving up. She didn't endlessly question "Why me?" Instead, she remained serene with an unclouded vision of healing.

Life After MS

It was hard for Darlene to pinpoint exactly when she became symptom-free; the process was slow and measured in tiny increments. Her best guess is that it was at least six years from when she started the diet, which places her full recovery at about 1980.

Over twenty years later, she doesn't consider herself to have MS. She eats carefully, still following the basic diet at home. She juices raw vegetables and wheatgrass and is careful to get enough of the essential fatty acids (omega-3, -6, and -9, found in fish and some vegetable oils like flaxseed, olive, sunflower, and safflower). When she is out, however, she can and will eat everything and not suffer any consequences. Three years ago, she told me that the only time she had a sense of still being afflicted by MS was when she was very sick with a high fever. Then she would feel a twinge of a symptom, usually the dizziness that first appeared. That is no longer the case and her healing has continued. The only food she has not added back is cantaloupe, although she reflected that she should try it again.

Darlene has left MS behind—it is not a part of her identity or her thoughts. A recent incident, when she ran into a young man she hadn't seen in years, highlighted how far she has come. Since she always liked him, she eagerly approached him to renew their acquaintance. He didn't recognize her at all. His shock at hearing her name was almost palpable. "But you were in a wheelchair," he said, still stunned. She had forgotten that he would still hold that image of her.

Darlene worried that she would not be able to recall enough of her MS experience to be really helpful in this book. She didn't realize how much it means to someone to know that it is possible to recover from such an extremely progressed case of MS.

Reflections

To my question of what was most beneficial in her healing, Darlene replied that beyond the diet, she feels ingesting an adequate amount of the essential oils was most important. She noted that it was important to her to get a balance of omega-3, -6, and -9 oils. Darlene also emphasized the importance of good digestion, including good elimination. The pains she suffered around her chest and heart were reflections of how closely connected MS is to the digestive system.

"Everyone is so different," she said with strong conviction, as if to counter the "one size fits all" approach of medicine. "It is crucial that you listen to your body in order to heal." She went on to say that she has lost the exquisite sensitivity she had to her body. When she was working on her healing, her body's reactions guided her to health. She strongly believes that the healing path out of the ravages of MS is unique to each person, and it is the individual's challenge to use the general guidelines and then listen to one's own body to find an individual solution.

Darlene also pointed out how important it is to believe in your treatment, whatever the context. "If you go to a doctor and he prescribes a medication, you have to believe it will work for it to be most effective." Research has documented her point that the placebo effect accounts for thirty percent improvement for just about any treatment modality. The same is certainly true for the diet treatment for MS. Through her belief in the diet, Darlene was able to hold to it for six months without any perceptible sign of improvement. If she hadn't been able to hold on despite the lack of visible progress, she might never have had the healing experience.

Darlene said she learned patience and discipline on her uncommon journey. Her healing was slow and measured in the smallest increments, at the same time demanding strict adherence. With the American diet moving farther from this healing way of eating, it becomes even more of a challenge to hold back and not indulge.

Darlene's experience underlines that body, mind, and soul are one. If our minds are full of negatives, then so are our bodies. This same wisdom is repeated in the many warnings about stress and what it does to our bodies. According to Darlene, living with deep faith and trust in God, she was free to move forward, unimpeded by her own negative thoughts and moods that would have blocked her healing path.

Darlene is an amazing woman. After having endured so much, her spirit is still open, fresh, and filled with love. That may be the most important lesson of all.

10

Patience and Persistence: Bryon

A disease process silently and insidiously establishes itself within our bodies, creating chaos and doing damage without as much as a ripple in our outer lives. It is often only in the later stages, with the appearance of some seemingly annoying symptom, that we even become aware that something is wrong. We are dumbfounded when we hear of friends or loved ones who go to the doctor with the complaint of back pain, only to be told, after an exploratory operation, that they are filled with cancer. It can take eight to ten years for a cancer tumor to grow large enough to be detected by our modern diagnostic equipment, a long time for the hidden disease to do its worst.

This is also the case with MS; the first event in the disease process occurs years before any manifestation or symptom. In some instances, by the time the first symptoms do appear, there are extensive lesions on the central nervous system.

It stands to reason that healing would also take time as the body tears down and repairs the ravages left by the disease. Just as the symptoms are not the whole of the problem, neither is the elimination of them all that needs to be accomplished in healing. Both our bodies and the disease process are much more complex than that.

Yet in our culture we expect instantaneous results, especially in the case of sickness and disease, a magic pill to return us to health. Too often, the suppression of symptoms is defined as a cure or health.

With the MS Recovery Diet, symptoms are not suppressed but diminish or recede when there has been sufficient healing. Parallel to the disease process, symptoms may be the last to disappear in healing as they were the last to manifest. Not enough is known about MS to describe exactly what needs to occur within our bodies before the person feels better and has functions restored. Like the disease itself, this is probably highly individual.

Bryon and Sharon's story illustrates how understanding this principle, along with a healthy dose of patience and persistence, paid off in complete recovery.

An American Family

"We're going on vacation later this month," Bryon told me on a hot August night as we sat at his kitchen table. Not a man given to showing his emotions, there was just a hint of a smile as he added, "Camping up in Wyoming. We're taking the girls," he said, referring to his two daughters, then ages five and seven. "I'm a little worried, though, that my knees will give me trouble if I carry the heavy pack."

I could envision Bryon forging ahead with a load almost equal to his own weight. That's the kind of man he is: determined and hardworking. He thrives on physical labor, his routine all summer working his landscaping business, as well as his own forty acres where he grows much of the family's food, including chickens and pigs. His lean, wiry build stretched over a six-foot frame gives no hint of the extent of his strength.

Bryon and his wife, Sharon, have built a nice life for themselves and their daughters, Audrey and Anna. Beyond working his own landscaping business, Bryon is a schoolteacher, as is Sharon. Everywhere you look in their house or on their land, there is clear evidence of a lot of hard work put into making their life as fruitful as it is.

There is no way that you would now know that Bryon has multiple sclerosis, certainly not from watching him or knowing all that he does. What you might notice is that he eats carefully, healthily, and if the proper food is not available, he will forgo eating. With his MS controlled, Bryon is symptom-free for the most part. His recovery is not to the point yet that he can eat the wrong foods with impunity. And he doesn't, for he has worked too hard to come this far to sabotage his progress by eating foods he knows will activate the MS.

It was during the summer of 1997 that Bryon first experienced strange things happening in his body. First, he experienced tightness in his forearms that he just couldn't shake off. Then tremors appeared from time to time and the left side of his face hurt, all with no apparent cause. Bryon's first response was to ignore it in hopes that it would just go away. He still tried to work through it when his legs began to feel weak, as if his muscles were worn out. It was a very busy time and he had a lot to do.

Sharon put into context just how busy they were. While their house was being built, they were staying in temporary quarters, running back and forth to supervise the progress. They had a two-year-old and a new baby at the time. More, Bryon was starting a new job that fall with the concomitant stress of the unfamiliar situation and the extra work of setting up a classroom. Meanwhile, he had a lot of landscaping contracts. Both Bryon and Sharon reflect that the extra stress at that particular time might have contributed to activating the disease.

All of these varied symptoms would come and go with no apparent trigger. However, one thing was constant: Bryon's loss of strength and energy in the heat. With all this happening, he was pushed beyond denial.

Medical Odyssey

"He told me that it was all in my head," Bryon said of his first visit to a neurologist. "And for a week after that, I really wondered if I was crazy." He laughed and gave a snort of disgust. This same thing happens to many people with MS, delaying their diagnosis. Bryon took action; he complained and received a letter of apology from the doctor.

The symptoms continued to plague Bryon with increasing frequency. His family doctor was of no help, so Bryon scheduled himself for an appointment with a university hospital neurologist.

"This guy is at least a decent human being, though he doesn't claim any expertise in regard to MS," Bryon said. The second neurologist gave credence to Bryon's symptoms and arranged for Bryon to see him when he was having trouble. A battery of tests ruled out other possible causes, including a brain tumor and Lyme disease. Multiple sclerosis was always mentioned, but no firm diagnosis was made, even though the MRI showed lesions on the white matter of the brain.

This left Bryon in limbo. Worse than not knowing the name for what he had, he had no idea what to do about all the increasing health problems he was facing. The only tangible help he had received was some medication to dull the pain in his face.

Decision and Denial

Sharon talks candidly of her preference for denial. Multiple sclerosis is such a debilitating, frightening disease that she held on to the hope that Bryon's problem was really something else. Along with this, she believed in conventional medicine—that physicians had the power to diagnose and that they would be able to offer some treatment.

At first, Sharon was terrified that Bryon had something fatal. The image loomed in her mind of her raising their two daughters alone or with Bryon incapacitated. Ruling out other more fatal diseases did ease her mind some. Either way, the future looked bleak.

The possible reality of MS became vivid after a meeting with a couple in their fifties, the husband wheelchair-bound. The man, though physically disabled, suffered neither cognitive problems nor the fatigue often associated with MS. An M.D. himself, he was able to pursue his career as a researcher. What struck Sharon was how unhappy and bitter the wife was. "I should take you aside and tell you what it is really like to live with MS," she said to Sharon as her husband was describing his life.

"All I could think was that I didn't want us to go that route," Sharon said, with strong conviction at the memory of that meeting.

Bryon more readily accepted the reality of the disease. Through his reading and knowing a friend with MS, Bryon became convinced that he did indeed have multiple sclerosis. He had watched this friend recover using the diet treatment and decided he had nothing to lose and a lot to gain by embarking on the same path. So, with no real guidance from the medical establishment, Bryon made a diagnosis and began the diet and nutritional treatment. Balancing her denial against all the evidence pointing to MS, Sharon made the same commitment to the alternative treatment.

A Leap of Faith

Bryon stayed on a modified Swank diet for one year without getting any better. Instead, he got worse.

"How did you do it?"

"It was all we had. We had nothing to lose," Sharon replied. "We'd seen it work," they both confirmed.

Bryon recalled how Sharon would weigh the almonds she packed in his lunch to make sure he wouldn't ingest too much fat. Under the Swank diet, the focus is to keep saturated fat to a minimum and take in an ample amount of the essential fatty acids. Bryon also eliminated dairy products and took some supplements at this time. "I didn't waver from that diet for one whole year," Bryon said with some pride. The delay in symptom reduction was probably because there was some other healing that had to take place first within his body, before the more evident symptom relief appeared.

"The worst moment was when I was in the backyard trying to put a swing set together for the girls," Bryon recalls. "I couldn't even hold a tool. Hammers and screwdrivers just flew out of my hands." The combination of the tremors, muscle spasms, sharp pains in his back, weakness, and the heat had taken everything out of him.

At the school where he worked, Bryon sometimes had to hold on to the walls to walk, he'd drop things that he was holding, and his vision blurred. He'd come home exhausted and sleep through dinner. Sharon recalls how disorganized and confused Bryon would be and described how she tried to compensate by making lists and calling him at school. "I'd fall out of chairs that I was sitting in," Bryon said with a chuckle. Time and recovery allow him to be amused now.

Sharon recounted that recently Bryon remembered something the kids had done that she had forgotten—a sharp contrast to that difficult time. She added that she had always prided herself on her good memory.

Their leap of faith paid off; after a year, Bryon started getting better. Bryon's symptoms were fewer and farther between. The cognitive problems faded, leaving miscellaneous hit-and-run physical symptoms.

Medical Odyssey, Part 2

Still with nothing firm from conventional medicine, Bryon and Sharon went to the Mayo Clinic. Again, other diseases were ruled out and again multiple sclerosis was often mentioned, but no firm diagnosis was made and no treatment prescribed.

Bryon also returned to the university neurologist. A new MRI revealed that some of Bryon's previous lesions had shrunk or disappeared. Bryon tried to tell the doctor about the diet treatment, but the man wasn't interested.

Undeterred and determined, Bryon and Sharon continued to modify Bryon's diet and lifestyle.

Bryon's reading and talking to other people with MS brought to his attention the factors of food sensitivities and allergies as a contributing factor to MS. Following up on that, Bryon had an ELISA test to identify his particular sensitivities. The ELISA test is only 80 percent accurate; foods that have been recently consumed are more likely to test positive, whereas people will not test sensitive to foods that have been eliminated. The immune reaction fades over time, which is why rotating foods is so effective, though it is important to bear in mind that any food that was once a trigger has the potential to cause reactions if eaten too often or in too large a quantity. Bryon's ELISA test showed no reaction to dairy, which he hadn't consumed for a long time, so he tested it by eating half of an ice cream sandwich. "I spent the next forty-eight hours in MS hell." He described the violent neck spasm, which caused his head to hit the window in his car. Bryon didn't find the test particularly helpful. He finds listening to his own body much more helpful than the tests.

By trial and error, Bryon learned what he could and couldn't eat without activating his MS. Still, with so many sweets lying around in the teacher's lounge, it was inevitable that he would fall prey to his sweet tooth.

"Did you pay with symptoms?" I asked.

"I always pay," Bryon replied. After a thoughtful pause, he said, "Lately, I've come to realize it just isn't worth it."

When Bryon eliminated gluten from his diet, he experienced the quickest and biggest jump in progress. With the establishment of a diet free of dairy and gluten, the two foods groups that seem to cause people with MS the most trouble, Bryon could maintain himself symptom-free most of the time. An occasional buzz of numbness and tingling or a slight sharp spasm might occur, he found, usually with a traceable trigger, though sometimes no cause could be identified.

Teamwork

Food is at the very heart of the MS treatment, so in Bryon's case, his recovery is very much the result of teamwork. Sharon, as the cook, is as involved with the MS and the treatment as Bryon. She reads all the literature about the diet, searches for tasty and varied recipes, scrutinizes all the labels, and prepares the meals. The combination of Bryon's naturally fast metabolism and the amount of strenuous work he does presents a challenge to come up with sufficient volume and calories to satisfy him. Bryon remarked that he has to eat all day to consume enough of the low-calorie nutrient-dense foods that are allowed in the diet.

Not being a cook is also a hindrance. Bryon does not just naturally know what is in various foods that are presented to him when he is out. Under Sharon's tutelage, he is learning more about food preparation, both methods and ingredients.

Menu planning is difficult for Sharon. When she decides what foods to prepare, she doesn't have the instant feedback or the memory of reactions to one food or another. She has to rely on Bryon to tell her.

Though Sharon and the girls don't follow the MS diet completely, the whole family is very aware of healthy eating. The girls, having picked up on what their father can and cannot eat, have taken the role of food police. "Daddy, you're not supposed to eat that," they conscientiously remind him.

Bryon acknowledges how wonderful Sharon has been through all this. She dismisses it with, "We're in this together." When someone in the family has MS, everyone is affected.

Bryon's recovery is a wonderful gift to his girls. They have a childhood free from worry and responsibility for a parent's illness, free from being limited about where they can go and what they can do as a family, and free to grow up at their own pace.

Maintaining Recovery

Dairy and animal fats proved to be Bryon's most troublesome foods. Sugar itself didn't bother him, he discovered, but the sugar in his beloved chocolate was usually combined with fat. Now, years later, he still will not eat those prohibited foods. He tries not to eat processed foods and has a large garden where they grow organic fruits and vegetables.

Now that he has cleared up his symptoms, Bryon has found that he can eat in moderation most everything else that was once a problem for him, even gluten. He finds that careful rotation is the key.

Fruits, vegetables, and lean meat make him feel better and he continues to follow the basic guidelines of his diet. For supplements, Bryon takes a multivitamin, calcium, vitamins D and E, as well as an aspirin. He still feels more vulnerable in fall and spring, something that Dr. Swank mentions, but never explains. Bryon feels it may be the change in sunlight. Though he often gets too busy to exercise, Bryon does feel that it helps him. He is very careful not to get fatigued, saying that when he does, it takes five or six days to recover.

When he does ingest something that triggers symptoms, all Bryon feels is a little buzzing (numbness/tingling and other odd sensations of MS) that is gone in eight hours. He contrasts this to the past when symptoms went on for days on end. He says he still may get a twinge or two, but in general, the disease's impact is very minor.

A Different Lifestyle

Bryon says that multiple sclerosis has made him appreciate every day. Life is more precious and valuable to him now. Beyond that, he feels that his character has deepened and he has become more spiritual. By forcing Bryon to live more slowly and more simply, MS has also brought him greater happiness.

Throughout this journey through sickness and back to health, neither Bryon nor Sharon ever took the path of self-pity. Nor did Sharon ever feel it wasn't her problem as well as Bryon's. Bryon never wavered in his determination to take care of his precious family. That, perhaps, is their testament to love.

As for the future, both see it full of new challenges and dreams of what they would like to do. Bryon wants to enlarge his gardens and do more extensive farming on his forty acres. Any thoughts about MS, or the impact the disease might have, do not concern him at all when he plans his future.

"MS is just not part of our lives anymore," Sharon explains. "We don't live with an awareness of it every day."

"It is about living a healthy life and eating carefully. But even the diet becomes second nature," Bryon said.

He wishes that the medical establishment would open its mind to diet as a treatment for MS. His decent guy, the university neurologist, has come around recently about gluten and the impact of diet on the disease, since his partner has gluten intolerance. That is just one small step.

When I mentioned a neighbor of Bryon's with MS who has reached the stage of total disability, he just shakes his head sadly that she won't give the Recovery Diet a chance.

11

Drugs and the MS Recovery Diet: Ruth

When I am contacted for the first time by someone diagnosed with MS, the person often asks, "What about taking one of the CRAB drugs with this treatment?" My answer is that the point of intervention for the Recovery Diet and for the drugs is different and they do not overlap or interfere with the actions of each other. The drugs act on the activated immune cells already in the central nervous system, and the diet prevents the immune system from activating in the first place.

About six years ago, I talked to Melanie, who had been diagnosed two years earlier and was taking Copaxone. She was still troubled by symptoms and open to the diet/nutritional treatment, which she immediately embraced. I ran into her not long ago, glowing and the picture of health. "The diet is wonderful," she exclaimed after telling me how she had shared the information with a recently diagnosed woman. "I still take Copaxone, however, just in case," she added.

It is up to each person with MS to make his or her own health decisions, and each individual has his or her own beliefs about conventional medicine. Ruth's story illustrates the many possibilities to take maximum advantage of whatever treatment is deemed helpful along the healing path.

Prepared for the Worst

Ruth and her husband, Chuck, run a family gourmet pie business in a historic bank building. Conveniently close, they live on the second floor.

Ruth, a little package of determined energy, came bounding down the stairs in answer to the bell. My eyes fastened on the electric chairlift attached to the wall tracing up the long flight of stairs. "Do you use this?" I asked, confused.

Ruth smiled, knocking off more years from her already youthful appearance. "Yes, after I go grocery shopping, I put one bag on the lift and carry the other upstairs," she replied. I followed her up the stairs as she added, "Of course, there are the times when my nephew's kids come over and ride the chairlift." She turned to me and said, "They love to come to Aunt Ruth's house."

So much for disability, I thought, as I continued to follow her up the stairs and into her attractive apartment. Ruth pointed out her doll collection, which extended into their bedroom, some even perched on Chuck's gun case.

Like her apartment, Ruth presented a unique mixture; she was conservatively dressed in taupe linen slacks and blouse, yet sported short spiked hair lightened to blond. Every so often in our conversation, popping out from her serious, driving nature, there emerged a delightful pluckishness and self-deprecating humor. Feeling quite at home, I settled in, eager to hear this intriguing woman's story.

"I also have an electric wheelchair and a deluxe scooter, which we call the Cadillac." She picked up the conversation where we had left it on the stairs. "When the kids come over, I let them take the chair and scooter out to the alley, where they have races."

I must have looked perplexed, because Ruth went on to explain what had transpired after she was diagnosed with MS. She had been losing her ability to walk. Right after she was diagnosed, she was given literature about the ABC drugs, so that she could pick one. She chose Copaxone because in the literature it was reported to have the fewest side effects. "Having flu symptoms two or three days a week as a side effect doesn't sound like much of a treatment to me," she said in wry commentary. Ruth was also advised to take it easy, not do much, and get rid of stress.

Following these orders, her legs worsened and seemed to weigh a ton, her back tingled and spasmed, and she had cognitive problems, especially in thinking and memory. Adding more misery, without her being at work, the business suffered. Beyond that, she suffered from the overwhelming MS fatigue.

Ruth says that she read all the literature put out by the National Multiple Sclerosis Society, which paints a very bleak picture. Learning about all the problems of MS with no solution, and seeing all the advertisements for wheelchairs, scooters, and mechanical aides, Ruth felt pretty depressed.

Though she had one scary reaction to the Copaxone in which she thought she was having a heart attack, she generally tolerated it. Beyond the Copaxone, she took a drug to help her sleep through the pain in her legs and then another to help her wake up and function during the day.

Ruth bought her equipment and was prepared to meet her MS future.

After six months of following orders, Ruth decided she couldn't go on that way. "We go camping a lot, and I wasn't going to be 'Chuck's poor wife who has MS,' " Ruth explained. "I'm not going there, so I decided to fight it."

"There's fighting spirit in my family," she said, and proceeded to describe an aunt who held on for twenty-plus years, active, busy, doing, despite recurring breast cancer with many associated problems. Ruth's sister, who for a time became very ill and unstable, was able to strictly control her diet to contain the extreme symptoms of hypoglycemia. Ruth knew that diseases could be conquered.

A sister-in-law, Jolynn, from Chuck's large, supportive family, is a physician in family practice. Jolynn advised Ruth, "I have a patient who is doing very well with MS. You should contact her—I've already cleared it." She also told Ruth to read everything she could find on the disease. From Jolynn's patient, Ruth received a large box of reading material to use and return. Taking off from there, Ruth read extensively about the diet/nutritional treatment of MS.

It all made sense to Ruth. She believed that diet could make a difference and was committed to following the new course. She began strictly adhering to all the proscriptions of that program—no dairy, no legumes, no eggs, no yeast, no gluten, low fat, and low sugar. "I lost fifty pounds."

Even though she doesn't like to exercise, Ruth was determined to fulfill that recommendation as well. With the same pluckishness, the ever-resourceful Ruth signed up for a paper route. The mile-plus circuit of walking satisfied the requirement for physical activity while satisfying Ruth's need to work and be productive. She visited a health food store in a larger city some seventy miles from her small town on the high plains of South Dakota. As it turned out, the owner was another person who had beaten MS. He confirmed what she was doing and helped her to select some supplements.

With this program in place, Ruth's condition improved within three months.

Early on, the family had stopped for dinner in the city at a chain restaurant specializing in burgers and frozen custard. As they drove home, Ruth's heart began beating so hard that she thought she was having a heart attack. In excruciating pain, she had her husband take her to the emergency room, where the diagnosis was possible gallbladder problems. Ruth figured out later it was really a reaction to animal fat, which remains her biggest problem food.

She also discovered that dairy caused her problems. First she felt it in her sinuses, and then she wilted with MS fatigue. At that point, Ruth usually stopped and rested, but if she pushed it—"Nothing worked," in her words. Her legs felt like they weighed 900 pounds apiece, and her brain shut down. "What did two plus two equal? I didn't know, and I didn't have the energy to care," she added, about the times when she was in that state.

The diet worked wonderfully for her—giving her confidence and restoring all her abilities. After she was basically clear of all symptoms, Ruth experimented. "Not all the things she had eliminated as advised by the Recovery Diet actually affected me," she said. So she added them back. To her consternation, she gained all the weight back as well. In the end, she found only dairy and animal fat triggered her MS.

A Little History

As a daughter of a pastor, Ruth had learned the value of faith, work, and family love. Ruth jokingly refers to the "Frey Philosophy of Workaholics," which is "Ignore it, get to work, you'll forget it, and it will go away." So when as a sophomore in high school her legs became swollen, bright red, and painful, she kept working at her part-time job in the bowling alley café. The symptoms didn't go away and eventually she did seek medical attention. With the diagnosis of rheumatoid arthritis, Ruth received cortisone shots in the backs of her knees for the next year. Right after she was married, at age twenty-five, Ruth experienced strange symptoms in her back, sharp pains or odd sensations, which she attributed to a return of the arthritis. "They were both early MS attacks," she says in retrospect.

About nine years ago, MS began its more serious assault. When her feet began hurting, her legs started tingling, and her muscles became tight and painful, Ruth couldn't keep up her workload in the family business. That is not to say she didn't keep on trying, even to the extent that she would pass out. One time she fell from a chair and another time she pulled out her rotator cuff in her shoulder. Still in full denial, she made excuses and explained these incidents away—even though there were no precipitating factors she could blame. Eventually, these symptoms subsided.

A year or so later, Ruth had trouble with her eyes; specifically, her right eye was blurry. A week after this problem appeared, she lost sight in that eye. "You know, I kept going anyway," Ruth mused. "I could still do most things, except pour a cup of coffee and that I found funny, even then."

Her condition was diagnosed as macular degeneration, something with which she still contends. As it persisted, she had an MRI and her first experience with a neurologist, who diagnosed optic neuritis. "I got my first bad taste of neurologists." He never mentioned MS to her, even though it was the diagnosis in the report which Ruth, as an intelligent consumer, of course read. The neurologist treated her with IV steroids, which she had two more times after that.

About six months later, though her eye was better, Ruth felt tingling in the left side of her face, her legs weighed a ton, and she was passing out on occasion. She also experienced the symptom of having a bolt of electricity shoot through her.

Ruth admits that, given her druthers, she would have just kept going and tried to ignore it. But her doctor sister-in-law, Jolynn, was concerned and kept in close contact, urging Ruth to seek medical help. With Jolynn smoothing the way, Ruth consented to see another neurologist. "After three years of fooling around with this, the doctor diagnosed MS in ten minutes," Ruth said with disgust, "I don't know why they couldn't have made the diagnosis earlier. If not for Jolynn, I probably would have gone years with no diagnosis."

Ruth continued her commentary on neurologists, none of it flattering. This included complaints about her present neurologist, who never returns her calls.

Beyond Food

Ruth strongly believes that some intangibles have also greatly contributed to her success in beating MS. The first one she mentions is her belief in God, which sustains her in faith and hope. Her father, a clergyman, still plays a prominent role in her life as an example of Christian living and goodness.

With gratitude, Ruth cites her husband, daughter, mother, and older sister, Janice, for their unfailing support through all the rough times. Love has surrounded her, lifting her up and helping to keep her strong. Added to this core group are the rest of her and her husband's extended families, especially sister-in-law, Jolynn.

Work, always a source of enjoyment and value, gives Ruth purpose; not only in producing something, but also in the teamwork and relationships developed as people join together to make a livelihood. In Ruth's case, it is the gourmet pie business, which produces between 1,800 and 3,000 handmade pies a day. As she puts it, "Good people surround me, as together, we create, give purpose and meaning in our work."

"The diet is important, but it wouldn't work without the right attitude," Ruth explains. "With the right attitude, you'll do what you need to do to get better, no matter how hard it is." Along with this determination, it is important to believe in yourself and the possibility of health.

Ruth contrasts her MS with that of a man in her town who was diagnosed about the same time she was. He followed the conventional medical approach. "He has the worst attitude—bitter, angry, and asking why me," Ruth said sadly. "They think he will be in a nursing home by the end of the year. He is doing terribly." Ruth had tried to tell him there were things he could do to help fight his MS. He dismissed all of her suggestions.

The Gifts

Before her MS manifested itself in a big way, Ruth was on the fast track with her business. She worked long hours during the week and then traveled weekends to do promotions. Her husband was gone all week, selling and delivering pies, so there was little family life. Looking back, Ruth said that she left her then teenage daughter, Heather, on her own too much.

Thankfully, the MS made her stay home and be a better mother to Heather. Despite having health problems, Ruth enjoyed the closer relationship she and her daughter developed. "It showed me what's important and slowed me down to be where I was needed."

"MS makes you get in tune with yourself," Ruth mused. She described how she had to begin to pay more attention to her body, indeed, her whole self.

At Present

Ruth has stopped taking Copaxone, with no adverse results. As a matter of fact, she reports that she feels better. She and her husband quit the pie business after years of fulfilling and hard work.

She eats well, including a lot of fruits and vegetables in her diet. Since she doesn't particularly care for sweets and baked goods, they are rarely included in her meals. Wild game from her husband's hunting supplies her with the lean protein she needs. Ruth still is careful about eating dairy or animal fat. Though small amounts are now tolerated, they can still activate her MS.

Ruth takes some supplements, specifically lecithin (which she feels is very helpful), a multivitamin, CoQ10, vitamin K, calcium, and rose hips.

Exercise is still not her favorite. Showing her usual ingenuity and enterprise, Ruth acquired an old exercise table, which was popular in the seventies. This apparatus mechanically moves the legs up and down while it massages or jiggles the upper body. She uses it to get her blood moving.

As for her MS, Ruth generally doesn't think about it at all. She says, "Fatigue is at the back door if I'm not careful," and sometimes she is bothered by a twitch or two. She sums it up this way: "MS is not a bad disease at all. It is preferable to cancer or heart problems because it is controllable. It's there, once in a while a nuisance, but that's about all."

Free of MS symptoms, healthy, and energetic, Ruth is now free to pursue new dreams.

12

Struggling: Letia

It is nothing short of miraculous that after twenty-six years with MS, Letia can go days without symptoms. Unfortunately, she is not able to maintain these gains. Her story illustrates the incredible complexity of the disease, as well as the need for extensive research to discover the nuances of both the disease and, more important, the diet/nutritional treatment.

Since I originally wrote Letia's story, her life has taken many turns; she and her family have moved across country, and she has faced economic instability and all the stress and worry that accompany it. Letia's fast metabolism, which kept her in the enviable position of being thin despite what she ate, has become a liability. She struggles to follow the diet yet maintain a healthy weight. Letia fights to stay above a size 2.

Letia is inspiring in her spirit and continued efforts for health. Even though she has not had the same results as the others profiled in this book, she remains undaunted in her belief in the diet's effectiveness and hopeful that it can be developed so that she, too, can enjoy an everyday recovery. Here is her story.

Eating to Live

"Look at them, still eating away," my husband, Steve, said to Doyle as the four of us sat around our dining room table one cold February night.

Letia's husband, who had long since finished eating himself, looked thoughtfully at Letia and then me, before chuckling. Then, turning more serious, he said grimly, "She's hungry."

"I've become a predator in my own kitchen," Letia explained with her knack for turning a phrase. There is something elfin about her. Perhaps it is her long, lean frame, her fine features, but more than that, it is the mischievous glint in her eye and her ever-present wit. In her soft, lilting voice, funny phrases just roll off her tongue; she named the new housing development where she lives "Legoland" because of all the look-alike taupe-colored houses. "I'm constantly on the prowl for something to eat. My greatest fear is that I'm going to wake up a size two," she said as she reached for more food.

The irony is that our husbands are big, solidly built men who could stand to lose a few pounds. Letia and I are both tall and thin. No one would guess that by volume, we outeat them by far. The difference lies in the fact that they can still indulge in the typical American diet, while we cannot. In order to control our MS, we eat very healthily, albeit a lot.

Letia and Steve began cleaning up, my husband noting how Letia continued to nibble as she put the food away in containers. I took the opportunity to get some of Doyle's reactions and feelings about Letia's embarking on the diet/nutritional treatment for MS. "She hasn't made the full transition yet," he observed, motioning toward the many vegetable dishes that I had served that evening. "She is still struggling with her eating patterns."

Letia's difficulties truly illustrate the challenge that people with MS face before getting firmly on the healing path. Beyond just people with MS, diabetics, heart patients, and so many others also must change their way of eating to fight disease or maintain health. The typical American diet is getting farther and farther away from what is good or healthy for any of us.

Naturally thin, Letia used to indulge herself fully on the worst of American food without gaining weight, the only real measure our culture uses to evaluate our eating habits. She had a premium-ice-cream milk shake daily, as well as all the dairy, eggs, sugar, and junk food she wanted. Upon reflection, Letia says that she ate so much of these foods she could probably have qualified it as an "addictive allergy." Since she loves to cook and bake, she always had wonderful treats at her disposal, as well. To the envy of many women, I'm sure, Letia, at five-foot-seven, maintained herself in a size 8 eating this way.

Multiple Health Problems

Complicating the picture, MS is not Letia's only health problem, though it was the first to be diagnosed.

At twenty, her eyes were not tracking right. She saw an eye doctor who gave her glasses, and the symptom went away.

Seven years later, Letia experienced double vision and headaches. Her prescription was changed and again the symptoms eventually disappeared.

Letia was just shy of thirty when she had her first big attack. Over the course of weeks, the numbness in two fingers progressed to engulfing both of her hands, arms, chest, right side of her face, and back. At night her hands felt like they were on fire. Desperate for relief, Letia would tie a cold pack around them so she could sleep.

After several diagnoses, including a vitamin overdose and shellfish poisoning, MS was named as the culprit. Unfazed by the diagnosis, Letia just kept going; she was busy with college, her husband and his new business, and her house. Despite her best effort, denial didn't work for long; she had to nap every day.

After eight weeks, the symptoms had not abated. It took two years for her hands to get back to a tolerable level of functioning, fairly close to normal. Fortunately, the MS fatigue went away. "I remember what the neurologist told me, which has been helpful over the years," Letia recalled. "He said neurological disorders are not measured in days or weeks—they are measured in months and years."

Cheerily, Letia announces, "I'm a cesspool for autoimmunity." About fifteen years ago, while pregnant with her son, she developed thyroid problems (an autoimmune disorder, characterized by a person's own immune system attacking healthy tissue and causing damage), which necessitated removal of the left lobe. She began to take Synthroid. Then, ten years ago, at age thirty-six, Letia had increasing problems with intestinal distress. This led to the discovery that she had celiac disease, an autoimmune response to gluten in the small intestine. When she eliminated gluten from her diet, the digestive problems she was having immediately cleared up. Interestingly, her mother had also discovered herself to be gluten intolerant and, in retrospect, her grandmother also suffered with this. From that experience, Letia learned firsthand the importance of food and nutrition in health and healing. The restrictions didn't cramp Letia's love of treats. A master cook, she merely figured out how to make her favorite goodies gluten free—so cookies, pies, cakes, and breads were still her normal fare. Letia is very grateful that she discovered gluten to be a problem. "I don't know where my MS would be now if I hadn't given it up."

Added to these problems, Letia had been plagued with constant sinus infections, vaginal yeast infections, and urinary tract infections over the years. Since changing her diet, all of these problems have diminished.

After following the Recovery Diet for a couple of years, her thyroid levels also began to increase on their own and her medication was decreased accordingly. Now her own thyroid is supplying her adequately and she no longer takes any medication for it. Her medical doctor told her he didn't know what she was doing, but to keep doing it. Letia attributes her improved thyroid function to the diet.

Most recently, Letia has been diagnosed with restless leg syndrome, which she finds can be somewhat controlled by limiting her salt intake. Not being able to salt her food denies Letia of satisfaction in her taste experience, adding to her difficulty in maintaining the diet.

All during these intervening years, Letia's MS slowly worsened, until she could barely walk, or write with her dominant left hand, or had enough energy to accomplish much. Her MS is a case of heightened sensitivity. No one food sends Letia to MS hell; rather, she reacts to a wide variety of foods, each resulting in a finite symptom. It is the accumulation of reactions to many such foods that wreak havoc and also make it harder to control. Letia's fast metabolism and the need to eat a lot to maintain her weight also make her recovery difficult.

It's Never Too Late

Letia has had relapsing/remitting MS for twenty-six years, the attacks becoming more closely paced and the residual symptoms increasing in the last seven to ten years.

When her family moved to the Midwest from San Francisco three years ago, Letia began to go downhill, changing to secondary progressive MS. Walking had become so difficult, she dreaded having to take her son to the mall, even though with her handicap sticker she could park right in front of the store, shop there, return to the car, and drive the perimeter to park right in front of the next store. Usually, when she did venture out, she had to hold on to her husband, or a grocery cart. She hated having the very noticeable, telltale limp. Her left hand also stopped working, lost to weakness and lack of coordination, so she had to write checks and type on the keyboard using only two fingers. Her left arm also failed. Another symptom, extremely disruptive to Letia's sleep, was a continuous twitching and bouncing of her leg. As if this weren't enough, she had the horrible MS fatigue. Her medication, one of the ABC drugs, wasn't helping at all.

An acquaintance gave Letia the name of a physician practicing integrative medicine, who gave her my name as a source of information on MS. She called immediately and we set up a meeting at a local coffee shop. At my words, "You know, you don't have to suffer with these symptoms," Letia says I had her full attention.

Letia immediately decided to pursue the diet/nutritional approach, allocating a year's time to see a change. She got positive results almost immediately. "I went cold turkey on everything," Letia explained. Her improvement was so good, she would have Doyle stand on the porch to watch her run up the driveway to the house in sheer joy. Everything in her leg was connecting again. Friends visited soon after and for the first time, Letia could walk the entire mall with them. "The feedback was so quick," she mused.

"But it wasn't smart to cut out everything at once, and I wouldn't advise it," Letia said with conviction. "First, it is too much of a jolt on your digestive system, which is accustomed to a certain way of eating. It lets you know—indigestion, diarrhea, constipation, or whatever—it can punish. And second, you don't get to distinguish just how sensitive you are to the individual foods." Letia also found that she was left without having built up a repertoire of alternate foods to fill her stomach.

After that first burst of elation, Letia is now going through the painstaking task of discovering all the foods to which she is sensitized as well as the foods she needs to eat to maintain her progress and keep her satisfied. Because each person's body, disease, and the interaction of the two are unique, only Letia can make these discernments.

She took the ELISA test, which at eighty percent accuracy can give a good start on figuring out what foods to avoid. It is only a beginning point; the real work is up to the individual person. Letia has found that she reacts to grains of any kind.

"It's not an easy road," she emphasizes. "It's not convenient, not mainstream, and it's expensive to follow." This is true. More time is required for food preparation and even for grocery shopping—it is never safe to assume that odd ingredients haven't been added to any prepared food. Going out to eat isn't easy, for there are only a small percentage of restaurants, upper-end and expensive, that serve the kind of food needed. People with MS have to carefully select the menu item and find out how it is prepared, and then perhaps even give directions to the kitchen. This can sound ominous, but both Letia and I have found restaurant chefs to be wonderful about this.

"Some of my relatives think I'm crazy," Letia said with irritation. "They make dire predictions about my health, especially since I stopped taking the medication." She went on to explain that she had taken the drug Avonex for eight months, but it only made her symptoms worse. "There was no point in continuing it." Fortunately, her husband, son, and parents are totally behind her on pursuing the diet. When she tells her friends about the eating plan, she is met with mixed responses, some people incredulous that she would go against conventional medicine, others supportive of alternative approaches.

Letia has also incorporated exercise into her treatment regime by swimming four days a week. She finds that after swimming, her symptoms lessen. Exercise also seems to help whatever symptom she might be having to work through her body faster. "All systems get going with more normalcy when I exercise," Letia sums up.

It was a big day for Letia when she gave up her handicap sticker. "First I tried doing without it several times and my improvement was good enough that I could walk from a distant space and through the store as well." She hated to have to use the sticker, a visible sign of her condition. "People stay away from you because you have MS," she points out. "They are afraid you'll get worse, and they don't want to be around to see that."

In the future, Letia sees herself becoming symptom-free and maintaining that fine state. "But first," she says, "I have to stop pushing the envelope and fine-tune my diet."

The Road Less Traveled

Since Letia has a fast metabolism and reacts to a wide variety of foods, she faces the daunting task of having to completely change what she eats on a daily basis. Her constant hunger and weight loss reflect her being in an in-between state—not being able to eat the old foods, yet not having a new repertoire of replacement foods. As she states, "When they say that the diet is a lifestyle change, don't laugh it off."

The question arises: If most Americans had to give up fats, sugars, dairy, red meat, processed foods, and baked goods, would they know what to eat? How many vegetables can the average American name or identify? More important, how many have they eaten often enough to learn to like them? Much of what we eat is what we are accustomed to, so the natural tendency is to stick to the same old comfortable foods. That is Letia's dilemma.

During dinner at my house, Letia had confided that the previous week had not been a good one for her, marked by symptoms in both of her hands and legs, making walking and writing hard. "I pushed the envelope far too much," she said candidly. "I used an egg in baking and put cream in my coffee." She knows the cause-and-effect reaction all too well; it happens every time she eats the foods to which she is sensitive. The two weeks before that, during which she had eaten very carefully following her diet, she had the predictable result of having almost no symptoms.

Letia ate the vegetables I served with gusto, proudly announcing as she was leaving that she felt full for the first time in a long while. The next morning, Letia e-mailed that she was feeling wonderful again. In the following days, she integrated some of the new foods that I served, like collard greens and celery root. Not surprisingly, she continued to feel good and be almost symptom-free.

In the balance of deficits and excesses that feed the MS symptoms, it is not only important to eliminate those foods that harm, but also to include those that heal as well. "I understand now that we can both eat our way into MS and eat our way out of it," Letia summarized. With this new insight, she is turning to the produce department to discover foods that will not only fill the void, but also heal her. Protein, in the form of fish and fowl, is also important both for health and to feel fully satisfied.

Frustration

Letia says: "My frustration is huge with this diet, and while I saw many symptoms abate immediately, I am up and down weekly with symptoms. I often see no reason for my increase and can't pinpoint it on one food. This leads me to believe that I am very sensitive to many things. The truth is that we are running an experiment on ourselves because the medical profession is unwilling to do that for us in the diet department. They are very happy to run experiments on us with drugs, however."

Letia wants the readers to know that she is very much on the path to finding what really affects her and so far she is not anywhere near being symptom-free for prolonged periods. She gets to a symptom-free state, but can't maintain it. "I am very sensitive to many things and I firmly believe I will discover what they are and be symptom-free, as I have been when on this diet many times—just not for longer than a week at a time. But that is proof to me that MS is well within my control," Letia explains.

A Choice of Attitude

Letia's upbeat and determined personality has served her well all these years. She has always been fully immersed in life, busy and active despite her MS. Since starting on this healing path, Letia says she is now more open to new ideas and uses more analytical thinking. Her growing sense of control over the disease has increased her confidence and decreased her fear. While she has become more empathetic toward people's suffering, she also has become more critical of what others eat. "I'm also thinking more in gray and not so much in black and white," she adds.

Letia sees MS as happening wholly within her body's own systems. To her thinking, it is the result of a hereditary predisposition to sensitivities;

she no longer sees it as a disease. Rather, she states, MS is workable, controllable, and really a part of her. "Everybody has something—I no longer consider MS a big deal," she explains happily. Letia credits her husband with being wonderfully supportive throughout the years. This certainly showed as he talked about Letia and her MS. He is impressed with how much improvement she has made and is sympathetic to her struggles in establishing a new eating pattern. He views people with MS who are working on this diet/nutritional treatment as food pioneers, who might lead the way for other afflicted groups to find their healing path.

A true partner to Letia, Doyle now pretty much follows the MS diet himself. His experience underlines his belief in the future of nutritional treatments. Doyle says that recently, for the first year in many, he didn't get sick with bronchitis, attributing this to his changed diet. He says he feels better, healthier, with the added benefits of handling stress better and losing weight. With a tinge of amazement in his voice, he added that he no longer craves the bad foods he used to love.

Still Working on It

Letia has controlled her MS in that it has not progressed, and when it flares up she figures out what she is doing wrong and corrects it.

After one period in which her symptoms increased, Letia figured out the cause—sugar. She has a true sweet tooth which, combined with her ability to invent recipes that work around the diet, was the culprit. She found that sugar has many disguises and that artificial sweeteners and the sugars in fruits and other foods all had a cumulative effect, giving her symptoms. Once she realized this and corrected her diet, her symptoms have, for the most part, disappeared.

She traced another bad time to her supplements, especially the cranberry extract that she was taking to fight urinary tract infections. Also, she discovered several of her supplements to be rice based, a problem for her. She is highly sensitive to all grains and to fructose, among other things.

With so many restrictions due to multiple health problems, coupled with her fast metabolism and hunger, it is understandable that Letia has a hard time sticking to the diet. The good news is that when her symptoms do start to get bad, she figures out what she is doing wrong and stops eating those things. By reining herself in, she keeps her MS under control so that the disease is not progressing and, best of all, she still has symptom-free times.

Last words from Letia: "Sadly enough, after five years of this, my diet of choice—and one that would be easy for me to 'convert to'—is still Coke, pizza, and ice cream."

13

Catching MS Early: Carol

The airwaves are full of messages about the importance of early detection for the successful treatment of many diseases. This is also true for MS, from all treatment perspectives.

Always unique, MS often presents itself in fits and starts for unknown reasons. I suspect it is a matter of the balance between the relative strengths of the disease and the body in its ability to fight and repair. As time goes on, in a large percentage of cases, the MS takes an upper hand, ravaging at will. Interestingly, it is reported in the literature that in the later years the disease activity lessens, even becoming dormant. However, at that point, much damage has already been done. This progression adds to the mystery of MS.

It is well established by Swank in his research that there is a much better prognosis when treatment is begun in the first year. All other reports concur with this conclusion.

In contrast to Letia's case, where the number of trigger foods is great, Carol's early intervention enabled her to avoid the confounding puzzle of food sensitivities. With the simplest form of the diet, Swank's avoidance of saturated fat, she was able to heal.

Sitting across the table from Carol at a restaurant, where we had come for lunch after the interview, I marveled that she had no visible sign of MS. Indeed, quite the opposite. Gentle is the word that best captures Carol. Her prettiness needs no adornment; her blond hair is simply cut, her smooth complexion flows over fine features, and her clear brown eyes reflect interest and liveliness. Carol's serene countenance gives an impression of a young woman in her thirties, not a fifty-one-year-old. Adding to this, several years of yoga show in her good posture and easy movements. Certainly, this is not the picture of a woman who has MS.

Wanting to Help

"I'd be very happy to share my story in a book about MS; I think such a book could really help a lot of people," was Carol's immediate response to my request to profile her for this book. She then related that over the last almost twenty years, she had given information about her MS diet—the Swank diet—to about a hundred people. "Of course, I haven't been able to follow up on everyone, but the three people I know who followed the diet are now essentially symptom-free. All those folks that I know of who decided it was too extreme or that they couldn't give up some foods are now quite progressed in their disease," Carol said.

"I don't understand. When my MS was bad, I was so depressed and desperate to do anything. If the way out of MS was to only eat gruel, then I would have done just that," Carol explained. It was clear that she wanted to help others experience the same success that she had enjoyed, beating MS and living symptom-free.

First Symptoms

In the spring of 1984, Carol was teaching language arts at a middle school when one day her contact lenses seemed dirty and cloudy. She cleaned them, but the hazy vision remained.

She called her father, a pediatrician in a nearby town. Carol explained that her father must have known it was bad, because he had her meet him and a neurologist at the emergency room. Once there, she noticed that her father's hands were shaking.

The neurologist examined her optic nerve, pronouncing it pale, and then ordered a CAT scan. At that time the technology for MRIs was just being developed and was not widely used. He then told her that her condition might be MS. Carol was scared.

Almost as a foreshadowing, she recalled reading about MS when she was about ten. "I felt at the time that having MS would be the worst thing that could happen to a person." The idea of becoming disabled and dependent was abhorrent to her as a girl, and the memory stuck with her.

Carol was given a prescription for prednisone, which she described as turning her into a monster. Beyond having everything taste awful, she was mean and angry all the time. Fortunately, her vision cleared and she returned to normal after a few weeks.

Several months later, Carol experienced another visual disturbance, specifically blindness in her right eye. Along with this, she had Lhermitte's sign: if she bent her head so her chin touched her chest, electrical impulses shot up and down her spine. She went back to the doctor.

During her second round of prednisone, Carol reports that she was desperate to eat. All foods seemed bland to her and she couldn't get them strong enough to taste good, leaving her craving flavor.

In another incident, Carol lost all strength in her predominant left arm after taking a hot bath. This persisted for a while, presenting a challenge to her in the classroom. "I did all my chalk work before class by using my right arm to hold up my left. Then, when the students were present, I got very proficient with the overhead projector."

More insidious changes were chipping away at Carol's life. "I lost semantic memory, so that in every conversation I found myself unable to pull up a word that I wanted." This was especially cruel to Carol, a language arts teacher and budding author. That all-pervasive MS fatigue plagued her as well. "I felt like heavy wet blankets were tied around my bones that I had to drag around," is the way Carol describes the feeling. She also experienced weakness.

With the full weight of an official diagnosis along with her own worsening condition, Carol felt desperate. "I remember watching a Bruce Springsteen concert on TV. He was so energetic and full of life. I cried, thinking that I would never have that kind of energy again." With the fatigue, the symptoms, and the sad prognosis, "I felt that my life was coming to an end." Carol was just thirty-two at the time.

Adding to her depression was Carol's reading of society's attitudes, which kept her from sharing with others her struggle with MS. "I didn't want to be known as the woman with MS." Her writing career had just taken off and she feared public knowledge of her disease would prevent her from getting contracts to write books. Publishers would see giving an assignment to a person with MS as risky, fearing she would not be able to finish the work. Now a successful author, Carol no longer has that fear.

Feeling her life being eroded by the MS, shrouded in misery and fear, Carol turned to prayer. With all the emotion of the past attached to her memory, Carol's voice quivered as she repeated her prayer of so long ago. "Dear God, I know that you heal people spontaneously. I can't believe that is going to happen to me. I really don't know what I'm asking, but I need a miracle. I need a miracle that I can believe in."

Shortly thereafter, Carol's husband, Ed, was with a friend in a shopping mall. The friend wanted to get something in a GNC store, so Ed followed him in. One book on the shelf caught his eye: *Multiple Sclerosis: A*

Self-Help Guide to Its Management by Judy Graham. He bought the book and brought it home.

That book made all the difference in the world to Carol. She believes it was by divine grace that her husband found the book for her.

In December 1984, nine months after her first symptom appeared, Carol started the Swank diet, described in Judy Graham's book. Carol followed up by getting *The Multiple Sclerosis Diet Book* by Dr. Roy Swank and Barbara Brewer Dugan.

"Dr. Swank said that there is a 95 to 97 percent rate of recovery if the diet is started in the first year," Carol explained. She immediately committed to following the diet, even more strictly than required. The basic tenet of this regime is to reduce the amount of saturated fat to less than 15 grams a day.

All Carol ate for the first year and a half was grilled or broiled chicken breast cooked without the skin, plus fruits, vegetables, and whole grains. She paid a bakery extra to make her bread with safflower oil instead of butter or margarine. She took cod-liver oil in softgels and lecithin as supplements.

"After four months, I felt stronger, lighter," Carol said, then added, "Actually, I felt healthier than I ever had in my life."

Soon after Carol started her diet, she did lose her sight. Visual problems are common early symptoms, which in Carol's case receded; her sight was fully restored. That did not deter or discourage her from her course. "Dr. Swank says it takes four months before results can be seen," Carol said. Again she was given prednisone for a short period, as is the protocol, given the risks of this steroid, and gradually her sight returned.

With wonder in her voice, Carol recalled the beautiful spring day when she passed a field of green grasses. Her vision was returning. "My eyes just drank in the beauty. I could almost feel the colors healing my eyes."

Carol found that unlike many people with MS who are heat sensitive, she was cold sensitive. Each fall, especially on those days when the temperature and the barometer dropped, MS would rear its ugly head briefly.

In 1987, Carol had a big project at home, during which she pushed herself too far. The result was a patch of altered sensation on her back. Predictably, that went away with a reduction of her stress and fatigue.

Carol also found that by cutting out diet soda, the ghost symptoms of fall disappeared. Aspartame is often implicated in MS-like symptoms.

Carol has never had to go beyond Swank's prescription of low saturated fat (less than 15 grams a day) and high intake of the essential fatty acids, the oils, to control her MS.

A Valuable Lesson—Learned the Hard Way

As the years went by and Carol lived free of symptoms, she became more lax about her diet, eating a lot of things she hadn't before. She even dared to eat foods with high fat, including Mexican food.

In the fall of 1989, Carol's MS returned with a vengeance. Both of her legs felt like tree trunks, and she shuffled like a surgery patient. She was horrified. "This is it!" she told herself. "I'm not going downhill."

Carol returned to strictly following the diet and three weeks later she was again symptom-free. Carol has rarely strayed since.

Laughing at herself, Carol explained how she weaned herself from her favorite chocolate ambrosia pie. "Every time I looked at the pie, I'd superimpose an image of myself in a wheelchair on it." That killed her craving.

Spirit and Tenacity

Where do the courage, faith, determination, and discipline come from to take the healing path? Carol found previously unknown strengths from deep within.

She describes her childhood as happy and secure, in a town she remembers as idyllic. Good health had always been hers, except for the occasional migraine that began appearing after high school.

Her first marriage, which didn't last, produced her son. Her second marriage has been successful and happy. Her husband, Ed, told her early in her struggle against MS, "You do whatever you need to do, and I'll be right there with you."

More than just drawing on existing faith, the healing path also feeds and enriches it. Carol can still picture in her mind the scene on a bridge, crossing a river shortly after she began her diet. "I prayed, thanking God for MS because it brought me closer to Him. Then the car filled with an overpowering love and warmth."

Gratitude for her life, for her MS, and for her healing is constant in everything Carol does. She looks at the world with a clear vision and lives her life with gratitude and reverence.

She attributes her full functioning to Dr. Swank, even though she has never seen him. Because she began the diet so early in the course of her MS, the regulation of saturated fat and oil brought about her healing. She has not had to contend with other food sensitivities.

Carol said she's learned that she alone is responsible for her health. She takes action to care for her body, even when it goes against medical advice. For example, even though some spots on her skin were judged to be benign, she insisted that they be removed. As it turned out, they were basal cell carcinomas. Without anger or rancor, her expectations are not on medicine to take care of her, but on herself. "Doctors are just people who can make mistakes sometimes, and medical knowledge and technology have a long way to go," Carol said. It is up to each individual to learn all they can about their bodies and their particular health chal lenges. Her own neurologist is supportive of her diet and has even shared the Swank book with others.

Carol believes that eating right, exercising, and having a good outlook are crucial to good health.

Looking Ahead

Carol is comfortable and open about her MS now. She knows she has control and is not fearful about her disease resurging. As an act of faith, she and her husband bought a two-story colonial house eleven years ago. The stairs are not seen as a potential problem, but rather as a means for more exercise.

MS has deepened her spirituality—a source of joy and meaning—and she is grateful for that. "I find that I'm more empathic," Carol explained, tears filling her eyes. She described hearing a quadriplegic who spoke at a workshop she attended. "When she said her dream was to use her hands, I was right with her; in my mind I could very well be her." Carol's already big heart has grown a few sizes larger because of her struggles—that's a precious gift.

14

Gifts and Lessons

Living with a disease as confounding and complex as MS affects us in ways far beyond taking a pill to kill a bacterium or to correct a chemical imbalance; rather, it touches every aspect of our being. Surprisingly, we find ourselves better people for the experience. Here are our thoughts.

Ann—The State of My MS

Am I cured of multiple sclerosis? Not at all; nor am I in remission. My MS is still active, and may be for the rest of my life. Though I don't deliberately push it, I am still vulnerable, though increasingly less so, to the wrong foods. Too much fatigue or serious illness, as seen in my bout with cancer, doesn't faze me any longer. These occasional reactions serve to remind me of the presence and power of MS. At some time in the future, when my lesions have closed off, I hope a true remission can be mine. But I'm not there yet. I still have a very faint fuzziness in the bottom of my feet, which I've yet to get rid of. Part of the reason this remains is that I have not been as strict as I could be, and since this altered sensation is no bother I haven't pursued ridding myself of the last vestige. Or maybe, the remaining fuzziness in my feet is there to keep me honest in my eating and health habits.

Lessons Learned

The word *grateful* barely contains my feelings on the subject of my recovery—ecstatic, gleeful, thankful, and more. I have a new appreciation and awe of my body, which fought back the disease and returned to full functioning. I try not to take my body for granted, to honor and respect it, even to the point of dressing better.

My MS journey has been wonderful for my health. My cholesterol and blood pressure, like my weight, had been inching up in the higher ranges as I aged. Not anymore, thanks to the MS diet and an exercise regime that is now second nature to me.

Learning about my body, disease, and diet, I have come to understand how the American diet is disastrous to our health. In the name of pleasure and convenience, we put all kinds of harmful substances into our bodies, and sadder yet, in the name of weight reduction, we do equal damage. We deny our body's vital life-giving substances and, instead, expect them to perform on artificial chemicals and substances toxic to us. It is a tribute to our bodies that they do as well as they do, given how we treat them. But this abuse is taking its toll on our individual and national health, with the rise in diabetes, obesity, hypertension, autoimmune diseases, and other problems. Baby boomers, the first generation to experience fast and processed foods, are just now entering their later years, when health problems begin to surface. Who knows what medical conditions our great food experiment will engender in our children's generation when they come of age.

The often repeated truism is that healthy living is a lifestyle. I can confirm that. Several people have commented that they should live as I do, that everyone should after they learn the detail of what I do. I agree.

The healing path of MS has much in common with the proscriptions for people with diabetes, heart disease, and even cancer. Beyond food, it includes rest, exercise, and taking the time to find inner contentment. Stress is toxic to our well-being.

My new lifestyle is out of the mainstream. I can't mindlessly fill myself by eating fast food or convenience foods. Instead, I must prepare fresh, live food to eat with full awareness of what I am putting into my body and how it will nourish me. I can't run on nervous energy or will myself to keep going no matter what. I must listen to my body and honor the need for rest and retreat. My slower, more conscious way of life is replete with contentment and joy.

The Gifts of MS

MS has given me many gifts beyond good health and well-being. When I experienced my big MS attack, I had a full counseling practice in a psychiatric clinic, which I enjoyed. It was what I was educated and trained to do, and I was well compensated for it. It just wasn't my passion. The desire to write novels burned in me, but was relegated to being just a dream. I had to quit work due to MS, but as my health improved and my energy returned, I took advantage of the time and wrote. There is nothing better in life for me than to be in the flow of writing and creating. As a result of this gift of time, my first novel has just been published.

Even my "me" has been enriched by my MS journey. The disease became my teacher and I the student, learning patience, persistence, and discipline. In the quiet of my home during my dark hours, I also began to look inward and connect to my essence in a deeper, more meaningful way. Beyond that, I felt greater spirituality and the powers beyond mankind. I found greater faith and trust. I live in a different world now—seeing hardships as opportunities, simple things and experiences as gold, and love as the supreme human accomplishment.

MS can be controlled so that abilities can be reclaimed and disability avoided—that is the message. I hope that through this book, and through the many other voices trying to convey this good news, conventional wisdom will spread this to people with MS and beyond to the medical establishment and all the institutional structures of our society. I wish that all minds would be opened to new thoughts and ways of being, so our society can move forward in health and happiness.

Judi—Recovering

At the lowest ebb of my journey with MS, I wrote a poem titled "My Savage Lover." I felt that I was intimate with MS as lovers are intimate with each other—its presence was there beneath my skin every moment of my life. When I first fell in love with my husband, I thought of him all the time; I dressed in my best clothes for him, I visualized him going about his day when I wasn't with him, and eventually, I learned to surrender to my love for him completely. My surrender to MS was never a joyful fantasy, even though every action that I took was dictated by this insidious being. Rather, I felt taken over by this horrible abusive relationship from which I could find no respite.

But even in my darkest hours, I have managed to find an insatiable curiosity about learning lessons and receiving gifts from whatever life brought me. This particular quality has served me well. Through the long, slow decline of my health, there has been great gain in other ways—life skills I would perhaps have received only when I became an elderly woman. I have often joked with my friends that when we all become senior citizens, I will be way ahead of them.

In my later years, I will already know how to let go of my former busy self, and to know who I am within the larger scope of what it is to be a human being. I have already learned how to ask for help from others, how to put up with the impatience of younger, spry folks, and how to release impulses and dreams that I cannot follow through on. I know how to keep busy internally, even when my body ceases to obey me. I know that a bad spell may well be followed by a good one, and if not, I surrender as gracefully as I can. I have learned how to speak to physicians and how to consider their advice without surrendering my own inner authority to them.

I am well aware of the toll my poor health has taken on my children and my husband, and I have learned how to make space for their reactions to my rising and falling health. I have learned to let them have their own reactions without taking on their burdens as well as my own. I know the keen disappointment of missing the final pickup from college, or not being able to watch my daughter receive an award. All of these lessons and blank spaces in my life are very familiar to me. I believe I have already earned a master's degree in old age.

Now I am earning my degree in recovery. MS never was, nor will it ever be, the definition of who I am. I am a mother, a wife, a dancer, a therapist—the labels are many, but these are merely labels and only reflect what I do. They will never be who I am. Even when I thought that MS was going to shape the rest of my life in some unknown nightmarish way, this illness could never define who I really was and always have been.

If I had suffered a broken leg, would I let that physical ailment become synonymous with all of me? Not likely, because I would assume that my discomfort will not be for the rest of my life. To me, MS is now similar to having a broken leg. I might have to walk carefully when the cast is off, and I might not ever jump off a high ledge again, but in all the ways that really count I am still me, before, during, and after my leg is fully healed. And I don't need to rely on a doctor to advise me on how to remove the cast made out of MS symptoms. All I need is to manage my diet. On the Recovery Diet, I am remembering who I have always been. Fueled by my renewed physical capabilities, life looks pretty sweet. For me, time is flowing backward in terms of re-membering my body, but time is flowing forward toward my new future life as well, without the specter of MS clouding every dream.

I have covered a long distance to arrive at this moment when I can honestly say that I am grateful to MS for its many teachings. Not that I recommend anyone having MS as a teacher, but the disease has proven itself a masterful mentor for me. Life will go right on presenting pain and pleasure and ups and downs, before, during, and after recovery; but the lessons I have learned while crawling up the MS mountain for thirty-eight years are indelibly part of me now and I wouldn't have it any other way.

Mastery

My new instructor is recovery. I start my lessons first thing in the morning. I live in a clearing in the woods in the Catskills. It is summer now, and my windows are wide open to the world as it awakens around our house. As soon as I rise, I delight in the feeling of my feet between the sheets. Just as a limb returns with circulation from numbness, I experience the flow of awareness in all of my toes, up my formerly numb-dumb left leg and arm, and all through my trunk muscles. I do not check for the recurring pain and exhaustion that used to inform my entire day. Instead, I delight in the trickle of sensation inside of my right ear, my jaw, and the back of my head, which was shut down by an inflamed trigeminal nerve just months ago. The fluid rosy glow of body intelligence suffuses my whole body, head to toe, and I feel a grin spread over my face. My eyes are still closed, but my ears are opened to the Hallelujah Bird Chorus.

I have earned this kind of morning—and I am still dancing! Recently, I danced at my nephew's wedding. Although this has been my own unique journey, I am very aware of others who have had similar experiences to those of us profiled in this book. I want to share the opportunity for recovery with anyone who cares to join us.

I have been fortunate to have had many healers and teachers who have given me great gifts along my twisting path. These healing experiences might have come through a professional or a "chance" meeting, just as this book may have come to you. For me, meeting Ann was such a happy accident. This "random" event led to my taking the Recovery Diet seriously eighteen years after I had briefly tried an incomplete version of it once before. My renewed endeavor was based on a meeting with a like-minded woman, although we are in very different stages of dealing with MS.

The gift of recovery that I treasure most is sharing it with my husband, Richard. In 2007, we will have been married thirty-seven years. We met when I was sixteen, the same year that MS first blossomed within my body. He has walked beside me every step of my long journey with MS. He has walked behind me, pushing my wheelchair in occasional visits to museums or while navigating an airport. He finally purchased a lovely painting to hang above my closet door so that my eyes could rest there during my long days in bed. He bought me an excellent radio with a remote control so that I could stay connected by listening to the larger world outside of my small, circumscribed life. Richard had to put away, one by one, his hopes and dreams of our future together, leaving only the few that he could do, or even want to do, by himself.

Now we are taking out our mutual dreams again and watching them unfurl in the winds of change my recovery is bringing about. The idea that I can be a full participant in co-creating an organic homestead in our corner of the Catskills is exhilarating. If help is ever needed to walk from the pasture to the garden or from the barn to the house, we envision it will be because we have grown very old and lame together. It brings a wry smile to my face to imagine one day that Richard might lean on me as much as I might need to lean on him. I could never have made it this far without him by my side.

Final Thoughts

My mother, who died with MS ravaging her along with the virus that took her life, is continually in my thoughts. She was only sixty-nine when she died, and I already know that at that age I will be healthy in ways she didn't have the opportunity to discover. Barring unforeseen accidental circumstances, I shall undoubtedly live longer than she did. I am her death as it lives inside of me, and I am my life as she lives inside of me as well. Living in this duality of life and death requires us all to become masters of the human condition. One vehicle for my emerging mastery has been MS. Another one is my process of recovery. May the other 399,999+ souls in America, and the other hundreds of thousands worldwide, join me in this new dance with a body that no longer suffers from the effects of MS.

Conclusion: Add Your Story

There are many people around the country who, to varying degrees, have done well in keeping their MS at bay. Some of these people have had the benefit of knowing about the Recovery Diet, while others have discovered on their own the importance of food and diet in managing the disease. Each has found that greater health is not always a matter of looking into a test tube, taking a daily shot, or electing surgery. Rather, healing and a return to health can be as simple as listening to one's own body and following the wisdom found there.

We hope that you will add your own healing story to the ever-increasing number of people who have benefited from the MS Recovery Diet.

PART 3

The MS Recovery Diet Cookbook

15

Food Facts

The Recovery Diet can be plain or fancy—it is up to your palate and how you feel about cooking. Eating simply means minimal cooking using few other ingredients beyond the basics. By this strategy, you can boil, bake, broil, roast, grill, or fry with the appropriate oil, all vegetables, lean protein, and whatever starches you can tolerate. The natural flavors and variety of the foods can keep you not only well nourished, but also satisfied.

Another approach is to eat simply most of the time, but when you have a craving for chocolate cake, pizza, or pancakes, or whatever is your comfort food, use the recipes here that substitute no or low gluten, low glucose, and no eggs, legumes, or dairy ingredients, so there's less chance of your symptoms being triggered.

If you enjoy cooking, these recipes offer a wide variety of flavor combinations of appetizers, dips, salads, soups, entrées, desserts, and more from around the world. If fact, you will find as many interesting and delicious foods as are featured in many conventional cookbooks.

To begin your diet safely, make the recipes that call for fish or poultry (minus the skin) and vegetables (although some people cannot tolerate potatoes, corn, or fresh peas and green beans) your first choice. The oils that are listed in the recipes are all mono- or polyunsaturated oils.

Nuts and seeds, their oils and butters, are also safe to eat, as long as you rotate them. Through daily overindulgence of the same oils or nuts, you can sensitize yourself and develop symptoms again. The remedy, as always, is moderation and rotation. Remember, even these "safe" oils contain a small amount of saturated fat, so be careful of how much oil you consume in any given day. As stated in Chapter 2, it is recommended to keep total consumption of the essential fatty acids in the range of four to ten teaspoons a day for maximal health. And a reminder, no more than 15 grams of saturated fat should be ingested each day.

Also, flaxseed oil and hemp seed oil do not retain their full nutritional value if cooked over high heat. That is why the recipes that follow use either olive oil for savory dishes or sunflower seed oil for sweeter dishes. Canola, safflower, and sesame seed oils can be used in cooking, as well. Use flaxseed or hemp seed oil for salad dressing, or directly on pancakes or hot cereals in place of butter. Each oil has its own sweet, nutty flavor.

In the grain recipes, we have noted that amaranth, buckwheat, wild rice, quinoa, and millet are not true grains and should also be safe starch substitutes. Oatmeal, cornmeal, and rice do not contain gluten, but may be a symptom trigger for some of you and safe for most of you. You will see spelt flour listed as an ingredient in many baked goods. Kamut, spelt, and teff are low-gluten grains, but it might be wise to wait until your recovery is almost complete and you have come to know your body and its reactions before risking a serving of any gluten-containing foods. There is also a sourdough spelt bread recipe that would be wise to wait on—it doesn't use baker's yeast, but captures the wild yeast that floats in the air all around us.

Low-glucose substitutes found in many recipes—agave nectar, stevia, and xylitol—are all made from plants other than sugarcane. They may also be something to wait on, in case sugar in any form is a problem for you. Eating well is crucial to the diet/nutritional treatment, which means not just eliminating the foods that trigger symptoms, but also including the foods that help the body. The trick is to have enough variety in flavor and texture to keep you happy and satisfied. Do not be daunted by either the Recovery Diet or this cookbook. Use it to find the eating strategy that works best for you. As you work with the diet, remember to always follow our mantra: "Listen to your body."

Take several weeks to find reasonable substitutes for your usual fare, and have on hand healthy snacks (fruits and washed, cut vegetables) so you don't feel deprived. Once established, healthier eating habits will be easier to keep. At first, switch to fruits as a substitute for sweets, and add nuts or nut butter to add the satisfaction of good-for-you fat; enjoy combinations such as almond butter on apple slices. In time, even your craving for fruit may diminish. See the beginning of the dessert recipe section for ideas.

Easing into the diet applies if you have been a junk-food junkie. But if you are severely compromised and won't be able to discern if a particular food triggers your symptoms for quite a while, eliminate everything except lean proteins and vegetables right away, adding in the mono- and polyunsaturated fats.

Organic, Whole, and Fresh

We can't handle the typical American diet, which is damaging and stressful to our bodies in numerous ways. Processed foods, with their many additives, give us less usable energy and expose us to more possible triggers. It is also hard to decipher the long list of not easily identified ingredients. For example, modified food starch, found in many products, can be made of corn, wheat, dairy, and eggs, as well. Fast foods—well, we just don't want to go there.

It is much healthier and safer to eat organic, whole, and fresh foods. Farmers' markets are excellent sources of good, local foods which have not lost nutritional value as many foods do when they are shipped across the country and have been picked many days ago.

The challenge is to be aware of every bit of food that you put into your body, and the more you know about the source and content of that food, the better you can control exactly what you are eating.

Time and Patience

Take your time in adjusting to this new way of eating. Your taste buds are probably accustomed to a greater amount of fats and sweets and, at first, you may not find this new diet very satisfying. But in a week or two, you will begin to enjoy the more subtle flavors of the individual vegetables and fruits. They will gradually become exquisitely sweet-tasting to you. Poultry and fish will seem more flavorful once you are weaned from the fattier meats.

Typically, fats digest slowly, staving off hunger, and carbohydrates add bulk, giving a feeling of fullness. The Recovery Diet greatly reduces fats as well as the usual carbohydrate fillers like bread and pasta, so you have to find alternative ways of maintaining satiation. Eating a sufficient quantity of lean protein is essential. It is never a good idea to let yourself become hungry because that often leads to grabbing whatever is handy, usually snack foods laden with fat and sugar.

Caffeine, like sugar, is also addictive. Many people experience headaches when they try to stop having their daily caffeine, so wean yourself gradually. Caffeine is found not only in coffee, but also in tea, cola soft drinks, and chocolate. Swank makes the case for avoiding any foods or substances that will affect your nervous system as caffeine and alcohol do.

Depending on how much of a change you need to make in your diet, give yourself, your body, and your taste buds time to adjust; be patient and stick with it.

Substitutions

Cooking, especially baking, is essentially the art of combining ingredients in appropriate proportions to obtain the desired taste, form, and texture. Over the years, recipes have been devised to quantify the exact amounts of specific ingredients for a predictable outcome. There are those people for whom no recipe seems to work, and there are people who just throw things together until the mixture "looks or feels right," and then they get perfect results.

The recipes in this cookbook have been formulated using knowledge of the purpose and properties of a specific ingredient and replacing it with one or more other ingredients that can fulfill the same function. The chocolate cake recipe illustrates this process. Cakes are a combination of wet and dry ingredients. Alternative flours such as spelt work best with the grittier texture of rice flour. Potato starch flour is smooth and helps bind the batter, so that is added as well. Bananas are not only moist, but also help to bind, though they have a strong taste. Reducing the amount of banana and substituting applesauce or mashed sweet potato takes care of the underlying banana taste. These recipes may call for more baking powder and baking soda than are in conventional recipes. This is due to the fact that banana is acidic and will neutralize some of the leavening agents. You can substitute rice milk or nut milk, cup for cup, with cow's milk. Agave nectar (a low-glucose alternative sweetener derived from a type of cactus) is a good substitute for sugar, but you will need to reduce the amount you use by 25 percent in any recipe calling for ½ cup sugar or more (not necessary when using a few tablespoons at a time), and you will also need to lower the oven temperature, since it is heat-sensitive.

You can use oils in place of butter or shortening; some are more flavorful than others, so keep that in mind as you choose them. For instance, you can try a teaspoon of olive oil instead of butter in your mashed potatoes. But remember, each spoonful of sunflower, olive, safflower, walnut, or canola oil, no matter how good for you, also contains saturated fat, so you must factor in the additive effect.

Most reactions to food happen within a certain time frame, usually almost immediately, but there can also be several hours' delay. It is easiest to work with immediate responses, as they are self-evident. Others may not show up for some time. There is also a typical burnout time for the increase in symptoms to recede, which is within about six hours or so. The exception can be at night, when symptoms can appear at any time, perhaps because our metabolism slows down. You may get just a short buzz right after you eat, which will go away within minutes. A symptom will only disappear for good, of course, when you stop ingesting the trigger foods or when your body has healed; otherwise, you are at risk for that symptom becoming a constant.

Even if you precisely follow some of the recipes using low-gluten grains or low-glucose sweeteners, you may develop warning symptoms. We repeat: as soon as you are able to make the switch, eating mostly lean proteins and vegetables is the safest way to begin reaping the benefits of this diet. At the point when you are secure in your recovery, then you can begin more food experimentation. You will find that you will have become more conscious and aware when you eat, which will make it easier to identify which food triggered a symptom. As you use these recipes and become accustomed to working with these new ingredients, you will be able to modify your own recipes using these principles.

Have fun with the recipes and explore and play with new ways of cooking and eating.

Shopping List

When you are on the Recovery Diet, you will do most of your grocery shopping around the periphery of the market. If you notice, most stores are laid out with the fresh produce section along one side, and fish, meat, and poultry along the back edge. This is where the vast majority of your food will come from, rather than in the middle, where all the packaged, processed foods are found.

Buying fresh can mean that you will have little food in your pantry. However, to enjoy the full range of foods offered in this cookbook, you will need to visit a health food store. There you can find the staple ingredients to have on hand for making all your favorite dishes.

The following list will get you started:

Nuts and seeds: all kinds, except peanuts (a legume), raw or roasted, to eat as snacks. Also nuts and seeds made into butters; keep them refrigerated, as nuts go rancid easily.

Flours: brown and white rice, amaranth, buckwheat, millet, potato starch, spelt, and cornmeal. Flour can also be made from nuts (chestnuts, coconuts) and even flaxseed.

Cereals: millet, quinoa, kamut, rice, teff, oats (found to be non-gluten by the American Celiac Disease Alliance), corn, and rice. Cereals can be puffed, or cooked like porridge.

Alternative breads, pasta, and crackers: rice cakes; rice crackers; pasta from rice, corn, or other alternative grains; some breads made from nut flours.

Egg Replacer: this is a boxed dry mix of tapioca flour and potato starch flour that will add some cohesion to baked goods that normally require eggs and gluten.

Milks: almond, hazelnut, oat, or rice. Remember that soy is a legume.

Oils: flaxseed, sunflower, safflower, walnut, grape seed, canola, and olive. Try to get a mix of oils so that you have a balance of omega-3, omega-6, and omega-9 oils. Keep refrigerated after opening because oils become rancid easily.

Sweeteners: stevia (powdered or in a liquid concentrate), xylitol (try to get the kind made from birch sap rather than corn), or agave nectar (light or dark).

Note: Remember that each person's experience of MS is unique. Rice, corn, and oats are generally not problematic for most people, but some find that these foods can trigger symptoms. Listen to your body.

A Word About Eating Out

Traveling and eating in restaurants and outside of your own kitchen can be a challenge, as you can't always know what is in every dish you are served. When on the road, carry along a bag of food in case you are stuck in a place where there is nothing for you to eat. This is important, especially if you have a low tolerance for hunger.

As for restaurants, the more expensive ones tend to be safer, because they serve fresher foods and prepare them on-site. Some chains serve already-prepared foods and sauces, so the local management has no idea of the ingredients. Restaurants also use much more butter than they usually acknowledge. Most good establishments are cooperative about restrictions, especially since food allergies seem to be on the rise in this country. Chefs can be surprisingly wonderful about preparing something just for you. Simply pick out the menu item that you think will most likely work, then try to figure out the possible trouble ingredients in the dish and ask for a substitution if possible. This can be easier than listing all of your restrictions at once, which may sound overwhelming to the uninitiated. Ask for oil and vinegar on the side, as eggs are often used as a thickening agent in vinaigrette dressings.

When eating out, breakfasts can be tricky. Eat fruit on oatmeal if it is available, and bring your own sweetener in a little bottle in your pocket or purse. Home fries can also fill you up, and sometimes a short-order cook will be willing to give you the vegetable fillings usually offered within an omelet with your potatoes on the side. Ask if they can throw in some smoked salmon or lunchtime sandwich chicken or turkey on the grill instead of eggs and cheese. Thinking about rotation, try to avoid any more fats for the rest of the day, since most breakfast places won't likely be using a mono- or polyunsaturated oil.

At lunchtime, many places offer salads and salad plates, so ask for tuna with no mayonnaise or for extra veggies or fresh fruit in place of cottage cheese.

At all meals, order bottled water or juice instead of soda. For dinner, there are usually more choices and, therefore, you will have more ability to make substitutes that come with a given entrée. Look first at all the lean meat or fish dinners. Ask for no sauce and to make sure that nothing is cooked in butter, as you are allergic to dairy. That covers butter, cheese, and cream. Ask if you could have rice or a baked potato instead of the cheese-puff pastry that comes with an order of chicken, or extra vegetables from another entrée.

Once you make up your mind to stick to this diet, social eating while dining out can be managed with a little effort. If you must have a small meal because of the lack of choices at a restaurant that serves mainly pizza and pasta, order only the salad and promise yourself some of that leftover chicken and rice in your fridge when you get home. Skip having caffeine by ordering mint tea, or bring your own decaf tea bag with you. Add the sweetener you brought with you while others have their coffee and dessert. Remember that your body will be serving you with the sweetness of no symptoms as your delicious just deserts.

Living with the Recovery Diet works out better if you do not focus on what other people are eating, even to the extent of not looking at their plates or paying attention to what they order in restaurants. Nothing good comes from dwelling on the negatives of what you don't have or can't do; rather, be positive and embrace the foods you can eat.

Beverages

Miss having wine? Health food stores offer a variety of sparkling juices—cider, cherry, lemonade—and a sophisticated juice product in three wine colors and bottles called Amé.

Lemonade is refreshing on a hot day. In a blender, process freshly squeezed lemon juice with water, sweetener to taste, frozen or fresh raspberries (berries equal to one half the amount of lemon juice and water), and a teaspoon or so of dried cooking lavender. Strain the mixture, discarding raspberry seeds and lavender just before serving.

- For an everyday treat, you can put a small amount of juice in a glass of water.
- A pitcher of water with lemon slices and a little fresh mint is an elegant change for a nice dinner.
- Herbal iced tea mixed with a little juice is also refreshing.

Holidays

Thanksgiving: If you can manage preparing the turkey and stuffing, and maybe one pie or a soup, have everyone else bring the rest. Use alternative flour to thicken gravy; bake corn muffins and break up for stuffing; and make your own sweet potato or squash pie for dessert, using Egg Replacer, xylitol, and nut or rice milk.

Passover and Matzo Balls: Use Egg Replacer and cooked millet (see p. 293) with spices for matzo balls in your chicken soup. See p. 268 for potato pancakes. Make sesame cookies with unsweetened coconut for dessert, using no baking powder, 1½ teaspoons Egg Replacer, 2 tablespoons water, and extra flour and coconut to get the right texture for the dough.

Other Holidays or Gatherings: The usual special meals that your family loves might have to be improvised using your new cooking ingredients. If not, prepare the usual for your family and just make a few substitutions for yourself on the side. Or bring along your own one-dish soup or casserole (pasta with protein, for instance) to make it simple for others. Many people have dietary limitations, and if you don't make a fuss, others won't either. You can at least join in with others on the salad.

Helpful Tips for Saving Time

If you want to make an elegant, special dinner and don't have the stamina to cook for three hours at a time, consider the following ideas:

- Make anything that you can the day before, like desserts, soups, salad dressings, and dips.
- *Mise en place* is a French culinary term meaning having everything in place. Prepare in place whatever you can ahead of time, including gathering up all of your ingredients so that quick cooking is all that is left. Make the salad; cover with a damp cloth in the fridge. Chop the vegetables and meat, putting vegetables like potatoes in lemon ice water so they don't brown or covering with a damp cloth in the fridge. Squeeze a little lemon juice over fruit so that it doesn't brown.
- Consider your menu carefully to include some easy heat-and-serve items, especially if you have some dishes that take more time at the last minute. Casseroles take a while to heat up in the oven, soups can be put on extra-low settings to keep warm, and while people nibble on your crackers and dips or crudités, you can slip into the kitchen to stir or heat up the final things. The most important elements are fresh ingredients and good fellowship. Good food should be easy, not stressful. People are often surprised at how delicious your MS diet can be. And they will feel better themselves knowing they ate well and are the healthier for it.

- The art of being a good host or hostess is having a relaxed and good time yourself. It puts everyone else in a good, relaxed frame of mind. On or off the MS Recovery Diet, keep these recipes and tips in mind whenever you are sharing food with others.

One-Week Menu Plan

The following is a list of suggested menus for seven days, with the recipes found under the appropriate section of the cookbook in the next chapter. As you become accustomed to both the diet and the new way of cooking, you will be able to modify many of your old favorite recipes. These meals, however, can get you started.

MONDAY

Breakfast: Cream of rice cereal
Lunch: Salad with a lean protein (chicken, tuna, smoked salmon)
Dinner: Fish, Quinoa,* and roasted asparagus or broccoli

TUESDAY

Breakfast: Cream of millet or puffed millet cereal
Lunch: Burritos*
Dinner: Spicy Shrimp* with tomatoes, peppers, and brown rice

WEDNESDAY

Breakfast: Hot cornmeal mush
Lunch: Chicken or Turkey Soup* with rice or corn crackers
Dinner: Pasta with Puttanesca Tomato Sauce* (with ground meat) and salad

*Recipe included.

THURSDAY

Breakfast: Hot potatoes and chicken/turkey dogs

Lunch: Fish and Corn Chowder* with rice cakes

Dinner: Turkey Burgers with Shallots and Mushrooms,* Roasted Root Vegetables,* and Emilia's Greens with Dried Cranberries*

FRIDAY

Breakfast: Fried Corn Grits* with fruit syrup or agave nectar

Lunch: Mixed Vegetable Soup* with corn cakes and nut butter

Dinner: Asian-Style Stir-fry with Chicken and Vegetables* (one of the three varieties)

SATURDAY

Breakfast: Pancakes*

Lunch: Carrot and Ginger Soup*

Dinner: Roast Chicken*, Millet Risotto* or Risotto,* Sautéed Yellow and Green Summer Squash*

SUNDAY

Breakfast: Corn Muffins* or Apple Almond Scones*

Lunch: Butternut Squash Soup*

Dinner: Chili with Turkey and Cashew "Beans"* with rice

*Recipe included.

16

The Recipes

Snacks and Appetizers

Sometimes you need to indulge yourself so that you aren't tempted to go off the diet for good. That's why it's important to keep snacks around. The healthiest are fruits and vegetables, which you can eat raw. Keep cleaned, cut-up vegetables readily available in the refrigerator. You can also buy commercial snacks without gluten, eggs, dairy, saturated fats, yeast, and sugar at health food stores, though these foods are usually starchy and not deeply nourishing.

Satisfying snacks are usually salty, sweet, and crunchy. Corn chips (baked, not fried) with salsa (read all labels carefully for added sugar in its many forms) or guacamole make good appetizers. Rice crackers and rice cakes can be used with the dips and spreads that follow.

Rumaki

Makes 20–25 pieces

12 slices turkey bacon

12 organic chicken livers, cut in bite-size pieces

1 (8 oz.) can water chestnuts, drained

Wrap a slice of turkey bacon around a cut-up piece of chicken liver and a water chestnut. Secure with a wooden pick, then broil or grill about 12 minutes, or until the bacon is crisp and the livers are hot throughout. If they start to burn, place them on a lower rack or on a lower setting if your oven allows. On a grill, keep turning so that the rumaki cooks evenly. Allow 2–3 pieces per person.

Potato Skins

Baking potatoes

Oil of your choice

Salt, pepper, and seasonings such as paprika, onion, and garlic

Wash the potatoes, prick the skin, and bake them in a 375°F oven about 45 minutes.

Scoop out most of the flesh from the baked potatoes (the flesh can be saved and served as mashed potatoes for another meal). Brush oil on the remaining skins, inside and out, and flavor with salt, pepper, and other seasonings, as desired.

Bake the skins on a baking sheet until crispy. Reduce oven temperature to 350°F and bake about 20 minutes, or until crispy. Allow 1 whole potato skin per serving.

Fried Zucchini and Sage Leaves

Serves 4–6

3 small zucchini

1 cup fresh sage leaves

¾ cup white rice flour

¾ cup spelt flour

½ cup olive oil (or olive oil mixed with sunflower seed, canola, or safflower oil, although pure olive oil will taste the best)

Wash and dry the zucchini and whole sage leaves. Slice the zucchini into ⅛-inch-thick rounds; shake in a bag of mixed flours to coat. Coat the sage leaves in the same way.

Heat 2–3 inches of oil in a medium-large skillet until it spatters when a drop of water is flicked in. Shake off any extra flour and fry all of the zucchini in small batches, until golden brown, without crowding (so you don't lower the temperature of the oil). Then fry the sage leaves.

Drain on a paper towel and salt to taste. These will have absorbed a lot of oil, so eat sparingly!

Stuffed Squash Blossoms

Serves 4–6

12 squash blossoms, any variety

12 tablespoons of any of the recipes listed in "Dips and Spreads"

Cornmeal or brown rice flour seasoned with salt and pepper

Olive oil

Pick a dozen blossoms at their stem end when open in the morning, but before they wilt. They are traditionally stuffed with a cheese filling, but any of the dip or spread recipes (pp. 225–230) will substitute nicely.

Place about 1 tablespoon of filling inside each blossom. Twist the tips gently so they don't tear. Dip them in water and roll in the cornmeal mixture until well coated.

Heat 1 inch of oil in a skillet. Add the stuffed blossoms, turning gently to fry on all sides. Drain on a paper towel and serve hot as an appetizer, or float a few in a bowl of soup.

Grilled Scallops with Turkey Bacon

Serves 4

24 large dry sea scallops (check with butcher to make sure they are not artificially plumped with water)

Olive oil seasoned with minced fresh herbs (basil, thyme, rosemary, and/or flat-leaf parsley)

24 radicchio, kale, or Swiss chard leaves, washed and dried

12 slices turkey bacon

Cover the scallops in the seasoned oil and marinate in the refrigerator for a few hours. Preheat grill or broiler. Wrap each scallop with a leaf of washed and dried green.

Wrap each leaf-wrapped scallop with half a piece of turkey bacon. Secure with a *wet* wooden pick or place several on a *wet* skewer, to ensure the wood won't burn.

Grill or broil about 5 minutes, until the bacon is crispy. Turn as needed to cook on all sides. Don't overcook the scallops—they will get tough quickly.

Spicy Granola

Makes about 5 cups

½ cup sunflower seeds

½ cup pepitas (pumpkin seeds)

½ cup almonds

½ cup cashews

½ cup pecans

½ cup walnuts

2 cups puffed millet, rice, or corn

1 tablespoon salt

1 teaspoon curry powder

1 teaspoon Spike (a premixed seasoning; optional)

¼ teaspoon cayenne

½ teaspoon garlic powder

¼ teaspoon nutmeg

¼ teaspoon ground black pepper

¼ teaspoon ground allspice or cloves

¼ teaspoon cinnamon

2 tablespoons sunflower seed oil or other oil

4 tablespoons agave nectar, xylitol, or stevia, to taste

Optional additions:

¼ cup chopped dried fruits

2 tablespoons vegetable flakes

½ cup chopped chestnuts

Mix seeds, nuts, and cereal in a large bowl. Mix spices together in a small bowl. Heat the oil in a small saucepan. Add the spices and cook until spices smell hot and are barely roasted. Add the sweetener (nectar, xylitol, or stevia) and let simmer until the mixture bubbles slightly. Stir the spice mixture into the nut mixture.

Spread the granola onto a jelly roll pan (or any baking dish with shallow sides). Bake at 350°F for 30 minutes, stirring several times. Let cool. Add optional ingredients as desired. Store in an airtight container.

Dips and Spreads

Besides being great with crackers, chips, and raw vegetables, dips and spreads can also be used to stuff fish, to top casseroles instead of cheese, as a sauce for pasta, a garnish for soups, or added to salad dressing for new flavor combinations.

Asian Sunflower Seed Spread

Makes about ½ cup

1 cup sunflower seeds, soaked in water for at least 2 hours or overnight

⅛ cup poppy seeds

¼ cup sesame seeds

½ lemon, juiced

1–2 cloves garlic

1 tablespoon peeled and grated fresh ginger

1 teaspoon salt, or 1 tablespoon tamari or shoyu soy sauce (if it doesn't bother you)

1½ teaspoons tahini (ground sesame seeds)

1 teaspoon mirin (naturally sweet rice wine vinegar), or 1 teaspoon apple cider vinegar with a pinch of alternative sweetener, to taste

Spread the soaked sunflower seeds on a double layer of paper towels and let dry 20 minutes. Put all of the ingredients into a food processor and grind until a smooth paste forms. If the paste seems too thick for spreading, add a little more lemon juice, soy sauce, or vinegar. This spread can also be used on sushi rolls (see p. 322) in place of umeboshi paste.

Green Pesto

Makes about ½ cup

This makes enough for 1 pound of pasta (vegetable noodles or alternative grains). It is also terrific as a dip or spread, or mixed into cooked vegetables, or dropped into a plain soup (about 1 spoonful) as a garnish.

2 cups mixed fresh green herbs, such as basil, oregano (just the leaves, no stems), parsley, or cilantro (stems included)

½ cup pine nuts or a combination of any seeds and nuts

1–2 cloves garlic, peeled

Salt, to taste

½ cup good-quality virgin olive oil

Wash and pat dry the herbs with a towel. Put the herbs, nuts, garlic, and some salt into a food processor. Process, gradually adding the olive oil until smoothly blended. If the pesto seems too thick, add more oil. Toss with hot, cooked pasta until well coated.

Tip: You can make this green pesto when your herb garden is in season and freeze some in a sectioned ice-cube tray to be used when it is cold outside. Just pop one out whenever you need to add a little pizzazz to a soup or stew.

Red Pesto

Makes about ½ cup

There's enough pesto for 1 pound of pasta, but you can also serve it as a dip or spread.

1 cup fresh green herbs: basil, oregano (just the leaves, no stems), parsley, or cilantro (stems included)

⅓ cup oil- or water-packed sun-dried tomatoes

⅓ cup pine nuts or a combination of any seeds and nuts

1–2 cloves garlic, peeled

Salt, to taste

⅓ cup good-quality virgin olive oil

Wash and pat dry the herbs. Place all the ingredients except the oil in a food processor. Process, gradually adding the oil. If it seems too dry, add more oil. Toss with hot pasta, or bring the pesto to the coffee table as a dip or spread before dinner. May also be frozen for later use.

Olive, Artichoke Heart, and Sun-dried Tomato Tapenade

Makes about ½ cup

10 large sun-dried tomatoes

3 canned or jarred artichoke hearts

12 kalamata olives, pitted, or 1 can anchovies in oil or water, rinsed well

1 clove garlic, peeled

If dry, soak the sun-dried tomatoes in hot water until soft, or if they come packed in oil, just drain them. Squeeze moisture from the artichoke hearts. Mix all the ingredients in a food processor or blender until processed into a spread.

Guacamole

Makes about ½ cup

1 clove garlic, peeled

1 ripe avocado, peeled and pitted

Freshly squeezed lemon juice

¼ cup chopped cilantro or parsley

⅛ cup chopped red bell pepper

Salt, to taste

Crush the garlic and mash the avocado. Mix together and add lemon juice to taste. Add the cilantro and red pepper. Salt to taste.

Potato Garlic Mayonnaise

Makes about ½ cup

1 avocado, peeled and pitted

1 small (2-inch-diameter) potato, boiled

2 cloves garlic, peeled and finely chopped

⅓ cup olive oil

1–2 lemons, juiced

Salt and pepper, to taste

Mash all ingredients together, adding salt and pepper to taste. This is rich, so use sparingly.

Eggplant Dip or Baba Ghanoush

(if this nightshade agrees with you) *Makes about ½ cup*

1 large or 2 medium eggplants

½ cup tahini

2–3 cloves garlic

1 teaspoon salt

2–3 lemons, juiced

Freshly ground pepper or hot pepper sauce, to taste

Wash and prick the eggplant with a fork. Place on a baking sheet and bake in a 400°F oven about 45 minutes. When cool, cut each eggplant in half and scoop out the soft flesh. Blend with the remaining ingredients in a food processor or mash with a potato masher until smooth and creamy. Adjust flavor by adding more or less juice, garlic, or salt and pepper.

Roasted Garlic *(sweet and fun to eat)*

Wrap a head of garlic in aluminum foil and roast in a 300°F oven for 1 hour. A knife should easily pass through when done. Squeeze the garlic from the skins onto crackers.

Soups

Call these "rolling soups" because you can keep serving them for up to a week by storing a batch in the fridge and adding leftover proteins, vegetables, grains, or even casseroles, as desired. Start with fresh ingredients at the beginning of each week and reheat just the portion you will consume in one meal. All soups taste better after the first day, when the flavors have had more time to meld. If you are in a hurry, keeping soup on hand makes a quick complete meal at home or a hot lunch in a thermos for the job.

en or Turkey Soup

Serves 2–4

1 yellow or white onion, peeled and chopped

1–3 tablespoons oil

2 stalks celery, sliced, or ½ cup peeled and chopped celery root

2 carrots, washed and sliced (leaving unpeeled retains extra minerals and vitamins)

1 small parsnip, turnip, or rutabaga, washed and sliced (optional, but gives full flavor to the broth)

2 boneless, skinless chicken or turkey breasts (about 8 oz./person)

½ cup minced parsley (stems included)

1 teaspoon dried sage, rosemary and/or thyme, or 1 tablespoon if using fresh herbs

4 cups chicken or vegetable broth (can be made with bouillon cubes or paste)

1–2 cups additional water or broth, if desired (less liquid, for a more stew-like soup)

Salt, to taste

Other vegetable suggestions, all washed and sliced:

1 yellow summer squash or zucchini

Florets and soft part of stems from 2 stalks broccoli

1 cup mushrooms, sliced

(If using any cooked vegetables, add these at the end of the simmering process, just long enough to heat through.)

In a Dutch oven or large soup pot, sauté the onion in 2 tablespoons of the oil of your choice on medium heat, then add other vegetables in order of density. For instance, carrots are dense, mushrooms are not. Add extra oil as needed.

While the vegetables are softening, rinse the poultry and chop into bite-size chunks. Stir into vegetable mixture and cook until meat is lightly browned. Add the herbs. Add the broth and salt to taste. Bring to a slow boil and then turn down the heat to low. Simmer at least 1 hour over low heat. If you have a slow cooker, you can skip the sautéing and fill with all of the ingredients to simmer on the low setting all day long.

Tip: If you are too tired to prepare all of the vegetables at once, start by chopping just the dense ones. Put them in a glass bowl, cover, and put in the fridge. Sauté them later as you are chopping up the softer vegetables and meat. You have at least another hour to rest while the soup is cooking. Remember to take out just the amount you will be consuming the next day and reheat gently in a small saucepan. Add leftovers to the soup to keep increasing the variety of flavors as the week goes on.

Fish and Corn Chowder

Serves 2–4

1 yellow or white onion, sliced, and/or 2 leeks, white part only, washed carefully and peeled and sliced

3–4 small white potatoes, washed, peeled, and diced

2 stalks celery, sliced, or ½ cup peeled and chopped celery root

2–3 tablespoons oil

8 oz. per person of meaty fish (tilapia, salmon, cod, monkfish, etc.) or equivalent amount of tailings (pieces of fish cut away by butcher that cost less per pound)

2 cups mushrooms (optional)

1 teaspoon chopped garlic

½ cup washed and chopped parsley (leaves and stems)

1 teaspoon dried rosemary or thyme

2 cups fresh (cut off the cob) or frozen corn kernels (use carrots if corn is a trigger food)

¼ cup white cooking wine (optional)

2 cups bouillon-flavored water or vegetable broth

2 cups nut or rice milk

1 cup cooked cereal (optional)

Salt, to taste

¼ teaspoon ground nutmeg (optional)

In a Dutch oven or large soup pot, sauté the onion, potatoes, and celery in 2 tablespoons of oil over medium heat until onions are translucent and celery and potatoes are softening. Potatoes will stick because of their starch content, so keep stirring and add more oil if necessary.

Add the fish (removing all bones you can see and feel) and mushrooms. Add the garlic and herbs, both dried and fresh, and corn kernels. Add white wine (alcohol will evaporate leaving just the flavor). Add water flavored with bouillon or, especially nice if you like mushrooms, use mushroom broth.

Cook until the fish is cooked through and flakes apart into pieces. Lower heat and add milk; do not boil. Add cooked cereal and heat gently if you like thicker chowder. Salt to taste.

Add grated nutmeg on top of each serving just before bringing the bowls to the table.

Mixed Vegetable Soup

Serves 2–4

2–3 tablespoons oil

1 yellow or white onion, peeled and sliced

2 carrots, washed and sliced

2 stalks celery, sliced, or ½ cup peeled and chopped celery root

4 small potatoes, washed and chopped

Additional washed and chopped vegetables to consider: green or wax beans, zucchini or summer squash, broccoli, parsnips, turnips, rutabagas, fresh or frozen peas (only if you are not sensitive to fresh legumes)

6 large Roma or 8–10 plum tomatoes, washed and diced, or 1 (28 oz.) can diced or whole plum tomatoes

3–4 teaspoons fresh or dried herbs: any mixture of sage, parsley, thyme, oregano, basil, marjoram, garlic

Salt and pepper, to taste

¼ cup red cooking wine (optional)

2–3 cups vegetable broth, or water and bouillon cube (optional)

Heat the oil in a Dutch oven or large soup pot. Sauté the dense vegetables first until softened, then add fresh or canned tomatoes, soft vegetables, herbs, and salt and pepper. Add red wine, and the water and bouillon, if you are not using canned tomatoes with their juices, ar for at least 1 hour. Add more water or broth for a thinner soup, a stew.

If you have a slow cooker, you can add all the ingredients at once, with water to just cover the vegetables. Cook on low setting for several hours.

Carrot and Ginger Soup

Serves 2–4

1 yellow or white onion, peeled and sliced

1 tablespoon fresh ginger, peeled and thinly sliced or grated

2 tablespoons cooking oil

4–5 unpeeled large carrots, washed

1 cup orange juice, or ½ cup juice and ½ cup chicken broth if you don't want so much fruit

Salt, to taste

2 tablespoons almond butter (essential)

Sauté the onion and ginger in oil in a heavy-bottomed soup pot. (Freeze the remainder of the piece of ginger in a plastic bag and save for grating into another Asian-flavored meal.) Cut the carrots into coins and add to the pot. Add the orange juice or broth mixture and cook about 20 minutes, until carrots are soft. Add salt and the almond butter.

Use a stick blender to puree, or pour into a food processor to blend.

Carrot Soup with Mint

Serves 4–6

2 tablespoons cooking oil

1 medium yellow or white onion, peeled and sliced

6 cups vegetable broth, or water with bouillon

8 carrots, washed and chopped

2 teaspoons salt

¼ cup chopped fresh mint, or 2 teaspoons dried (you can open up a tea bag)

2 tablespoons agave nectar or xylitol, or stevia, to taste

Pour the oil into a medium-size soup pot over medium heat and sauté the onion about 5 minutes, until translucent. Add the broth and carrots and simmer about 30 minutes, until the carrots are soft. Puree in a food processor or with a stick blender. Add salt, mint, and sweetener; mix well and adjust to taste. If using fresh mint, pick some leaves to garnish each bowl.

Vichyssoise

Serves 4–6

1 cup chopped leeks (white parts only, well rinsed)

1 cup chopped white or yellow onion

2 tablespoons cooking oil

8 medium potatoes, washed and chopped

3 cloves garlic, peeled and minced

4 cups vegetable or chicken broth

2 cups sorrel or other tart green (watercress, arugula, or spinach), washed and drained

2–3 cups nut or rice milk

Salt and pepper, to taste

Fresh sage, rosemary, or parsley for garnish (optional)

Sauté the leeks and onion in oil in a large soup pot over medi heat until translucent. Add the potatoes and stir well. Add the garlic a enough broth to cover the vegetables, adding more water if necessary. Boil gently 15–20 minutes, until potatoes are just soft, testing with a fork.

Add the greens and cook about 5 more minutes, until wilted. Add 2 cups of nut or rice milk and puree with a stick blender or in a food processor to blend. Add more milk until desired consistency is reached. Add salt and pepper to taste.

Let cool to room temperature, refrigerate until chilled (in summer), or reheat gently (in winter). If you have fresh herbs, a sprig of sage, rosemary, or parsley makes a nice garnish for each bowl.

Mint and Zucchini Soup

Serves 2–4

1 red onion, peeled and chopped

1 cup chopped leeks (white part only, well washed)

2–3 tablespoons olive or other cooking oil

1 pound Idaho potatoes, washed, peeled, and diced

1 teaspoon salt

3 pounds zucchini, washed and diced

¼ cup mint leaves, washed and patted dry

¼ cup basil leaves, washed and patted dry

1 cup flat-leaf parsley, washed and patted dry

Salt and pepper, to taste

2 tablespoons olive oil (optional)

Sauté the onion and leeks in olive oil in a soup pot over medium heat until translucent. Add potatoes and stir 2 minutes. Add salt (about 1 teaspoon) and enough water to barely cover the potatoes. Simmer over medium-low heat 10 minutes. Add the zucchini and ½ cup water and simmer about 5 minutes, until zucchini is cooked through. Add the fresh herbs and salt and pepper to taste.

Remove from the heat and puree with a stick blender or in a food processor. If too thick, add up to 2 tablespoons olive oil. This soup should be eaten right away.

Variation: This recipe is best if fresh herbs are used, and others may be used in place of the basil and parsley: oregano, thyme, sage, and cilantro. Save some fresh mint leaves for a garnish.

Butternut Squash Soup

Serves 2–4

1 medium-large butternut squash

1 tablespoon cooking oil

1 large apple (any kind), cored and chopped

1 yellow or white onion, peeled and sliced

2–4 cups vegetable or chicken broth

Pinch ground nutmeg

Salt, to taste

1 teaspoon peeled and grated fresh ginger (optional)

Cut off the ends of the butternut squash and split in half lengthwise. Scoop out the seeds, peel off the skin with a vegetable peeler, and cut into small chunks. Sauté the squash in oil in a heavy-bottomed pot over medium-high heat.

Add the apple and onion and stir until the vegetables are beginning to soften. Add more oil if needed. Add enough of the broth to cover the vegetables.

Cover the pot and simmer over low heat about 20 minutes, or until cooked and soft. Puree with a stick blender, or put in a food processor to blend. Add nutmeg and salt when done.

Note: Butternut squash has a thinner skin than other hard squashes and so it is easier to peel. Cheese pumpkins or other squash can be used here as well (see Pumpkin Soup, below). If you use a harder squash, split it in half, remove the seeds, and bake it in a 350°F oven in a pan with an inch of water until soft. When the pumpkin is cool, separate the flesh from the peel and add to the cooked onion and apple as on page 238.

Tip: If you add turkey or chicken sausage slices after the soup is blended, you have a complete meal. Heat gently until sausage is hot. You can also add 1 teaspoon grated ginger, which is very good for digestion.

Pumpkin Soup

Makes at least 8 cups; exact yield depends on size of pumpkin

1 medium-large pumpkin (cheese pumpkins are great for cooking)

4 cups apple cider (or chicken broth if you are fructose-intolerant)

½ teaspoon cinnamon

½ teaspoon nutmeg

Salt, to taste

Split the pumpkin open and remove seeds. Cut the shell into 6-inch chunks. Place in a large soup pot, cover with water, and boil over high heat until the flesh is soft. Remove from the heat and, when cool, separate the flesh from the rind. The pumpkin can also be baked to remove the flesh (see preceding recipe).

Puree with a stick blender or in a food processor with cider or chicken broth until desired consistency is reached. Add spices and salt to taste.

Gazpacho with Pesto

Serves 4–6

This is so flavorful that a small cup or bowl can suffice for each person.

10–12 large sun-dried tomatoes

Juice of 2 oranges

2 tablespoons apple cider vinegar

1 teaspoon salt

2 cloves garlic, peeled

½ cup chopped red onion or scallions

½ cup pine nuts or mix of sunflower seeds and nuts

2 large fresh, ripe summer tomatoes, or 4 canned plum tomatoes (juice squeezed out by hand)

1 medium-size cucumber, zucchini, or yellow summer squash, washed and chopped

2 stalks celery, washed and chopped

½ cup sliced red or green bell pepper, washed and chopped

1¼ cups fresh herbs (a mixture of basil, parsley, cilantro, and/or oregano); a predominance of basil is traditional but not necessary)

Soak the sun-dried tomatoes in the orange juice and vinegar for 1 hour, or until soft. Put all of the ingredients into a food processor and blend until mixed but not completely smooth.

Place in the fridge for at least 1 hour or overnight to allow flavors to blend. Serve chilled. This is a great party dish, as it can be made in advance.

Salads

The two most important elements of the Recovery Diet are vegetables and lean protein. Some produce items release different nutrients when cooked than when eaten raw. Raw vegetables offer their enzymes to aid in digestion, but to keep foods varied, you should use a combination of both raw and cooked vegetables in your daily meal plans.

A word about the nightshade family of vegetables, which includes tomatoes, potatoes, peppers, and eggplants. These foods can be troublesome to a small percentage of people with rheumatoid arthritis and migraines and some who are simply allergic to them. Also, cucumbers often cause indigestion and should be avoided if they affect you this way; when pickled, or cooked like any summer squash, cucumbers may be much easier to digest.

Salads make a nice addition to any meal. Try matching the salad dressing with the flavors of your main course: a sesame oil–based dressing for a Chinese-style meal, and balsamic vinegar and olive oil with Italian food. This is just a partial list of the vegetables, nuts, fruits, and other foods that can be used to keep your salads interesting:

Lettuces and greens (mild, tart, soft, and crisp varieties)
Tomatoes
Cucumbers
Beets (grated raw or cooked)
Bell peppers (all colors)
Radishes (white, red, watermelon, and daikon)
Grated baby carrots or thinly sliced large carrots
Avocados
Leftover cooked vegetables, grains, or proteins
Walnuts, cashews, pecans, sunflower seeds
½ sliced apple or pear, grapes, oranges, kumquats, dried cranberries, other berries
Red onions, Walla Walla onions, Vidalia onions, or scallions
Mushrooms
Celery
Canned tuna, salmon, or shrimp, or other cooked protein

Country Garden Salad

If you are lucky enough to have access to fresh herbs in the summer, consider using half lettuce and arugula and half herb leaves, such as tarragon, oregano, marjoram, or lots of basil and parsley, and a little mint, as well. Dress with a drizzle of healthy oil and balsamic vinegar or a squeeze of fresh lemon juice and salt.

Hot Potato Salad with Turkey Bacon and Walnuts

6 cups arugula or mesclun (mixed baby greens—lettuces, spinach, and radicchio) and/or watercress, washed and spun dry

4 large yellow potatoes, washed and diced

4 oz. turkey bacon

1 cup walnut pieces

4 tablespoons salad oil

2 tablespoons balsamic vinegar

Place the greens in a salad bowl.

Boil the potatoes in water about 10 minutes, until cooked but still firm. Fry the turkey bacon in a small skillet or broil in a toaster oven about 3 minutes, until heated through.

Place all the ingredients in the salad bowl and toss with oil and vinegar. This salad can also stand at room temperature while you prepare other food.

Citrus Fruit Salad with Fennel or Avocado

Serves 4

2–3 large fennel bulbs with bottom removed, no stalks or feathery leaves

1 blood orange, peeled and sectioned

1 navel orange, peeled and sectioned

1 ruby red grapefruit, peeled and sectioned

Juice of ½ lemon

2 tablespoons salad oil

Salt, to taste

1 teaspoon dried oregano or thyme

For avocado salad:

1 large avocado, sliced

1 tablespoon poppy seed

Slice the fennel into a salad bowl and section citrus fruit over the bowl to catch all juices. There should be twice as much fennel as fruit. Toss with lemon juice, oil, and herbs. For avocado salad, there should be twice as much fruit as avocado. Add poppy seed to the dressing.

Blood oranges are tart and sweet and look gorgeous. Use them often in season.

Hot Cucumber Salad

Serves 4

Asian recipes often call for cooked cucumbers, which are more digestible.

1 tablespoon dark roasted sesame seed oil (essential)

2 tablespoons chopped walnuts, or sunflower seeds

1 cucumber, peeled, seeded, and finely diced

3 stalks celery, washed and thinly sliced

1 head romaine lettuce, washed and cut into 1-inch strips

Juice of 1 lemon

½ teaspoon dill weed

Salt and pepper, to taste

Heat the sesame oil in a large skillet or Dutch oven over medium heat and brown the nuts or seeds. Stir in the cucumber and celery and stir-fry 2 minutes. Add the romaine and sauté until wilted.

Remove from the heat and stir in the lemon juice and seasonings. Serve immediately Use this salad to accompany any Asian-style meal.

Beet Salad with Walnuts and Raspberries

Serves 4

6 small red beets, washed (save the tops for later to cook as you would any greens)

1 small red onion, sliced into very thin rounds

1 cup walnuts, toasted (heat on a tray in a toaster oven at 350°F for 10–12 minutes)

2 tablespoons sweetener (if using xylitol, dissolve in vinegar)

2 tablespoons balsamic vinegar

¼ cup fresh or thawed frozen raspberries

⅓ cup flat-leaf parsley, washed and chopped (stems included)

1 teaspoon salt

Place the beets in a saucepan, cover with water, and boil 40 minutes, or until soft when pricked with a fork. Rinse well in cold water until cool enough to handle. Remove the skins and cut into ¼-inch slices. (Wear rubber gloves if you don't want stained fingers.)

Boil the onions 3 minutes, or until translucent.

Mix together all the ingredients in a salad bowl and let stand for at least 30 minutes. Serve at room temperature, or refrigerate and serve chilled.

Carrot Salad

Serves 4

Wash and grate 3 or 4 large carrots by hand or with a grater blade in a food processor. (If you leave the peel on, you will have more nutrients. If you don't want any brown specks in the salad, then you should peel the carrots.) Squeeze some lemon juice and a teaspoon of salad oil over carrots, and salt to taste.

Variations:

Add any salad dressing, pp. 253–257.

Add chopped or grated apple, pear, seeds, or nuts.

Add 1 tablespoon caraway seed.

Add grated cabbage for coleslaw and use Potato Garlic Mayonnaise, p. 229.

Add 1 teaspoon cumin seed and ½ cup pitted, chopped olives for a Middle Eastern flair.

Wilted Spinach with Blood Oranges

Serves 4

1 pound fresh whole spinach or baby spinach leaves, washed and chopped

2 blood oranges, sliced into rounds with the peels cut away (navel oranges can be used instead)

¼ cup walnut pieces

¼ cup scallions or red onion, thinly sliced

1 clove garlic, minced

¼ cup pitted black olives, chopped (optional, but a tasty contrast to the oranges)

Olive or other salad oil

Balsamic vinegar

Salt, to taste

Heat the broiler. Let the spinach leaves stay wet after washing them carefully to remove all grit. In a pan with sides that can be placed under the broiler, put all ingredients except the oil, vinegar, and salt into the pan and mix well. Drizzle with the oil and vinegar and salt to taste.

Place under the broiler at a medium setting or on a slightly lower rack for just a few minutes, or until the spinach has just wilted. Watch carefully, as spinach and walnuts can burn quickly. Serve immediately. This is an elegant start to any meal.

Winter Salad

Serves 4

½ bunch kale, washed, stems minced, and leaves finely shredded

2 large carrots, washed and grated

¼ cup minced red onion

½ cup sunflower seeds

¼ cup dried cranberries (or raisins, currants, or other dried berries)

3 tablespoons salad oil

2 tablespoons balsamic vinegar

Salt and pepper, to taste

Place all the ingredients in a medium salad bowl and toss. Let the kale wilt in the dressing at room temperature at least 2 hours before serving.

Nat's Bay Shrimp Salad

Serves 4–6

6 washed butter lettuce leaves, left whole if small, if larger, torn into bite-size pieces

1 medium cucumber, peeled, halved lengthwise, seeded, and thinly sliced (if sensitive to cucumber, use 1 stalk celery instead, thinly sliced)

1 red or orange bell pepper, seeded and thinly sliced

1 pound precooked bay shrimp

Lemon Vinaigrette (p. 255)

2 tablespoons finely chopped fresh dill, or 1 tablespoon dried

Fresh dill or parsley sprigs (for garnish)

Arrange the lettuce on individual serving plates. Arrange the cucumber (or celery) and pepper slices and mound the shrimp on top.

In a small bowl, mix lemon vinaigrette with dill and, just before serving, drizzle the dressing on top of the shrimp and vegetables. Garnish with dill or parsley.

Mort's Potato, Anchovy, and Tuna Salad

Serves 4–6

1⅔ cups whole small potatoes or diced cold boiled potatoes

Lemon Vinaigrette (p. 255)

2 tablespoons finely chopped parsley (stems included)

1 clove garlic, finely chopped

3 cups packed arugula leaves, washed and spun dry

2 medium heads Belgian endive, washed, dried, and thinly sliced

1 (16.5 oz.) can tuna, drained and broken into coarse chunks

1 (2 oz.) can anchovies in oil or water, rinsed and separated

Freshly ground black pepper

Stir the potatoes with lemon vinaigrette, parsley, and garlic. Cover and marinate in the fridge at least 1 hour.

Before serving, fill each plate with a bed of arugula leaves. Add endives in the center. Mound the potatoes and chunks of tuna on top. Garnish with anchovies and black pepper.

Fresh Fish and Grapefruit Pasta Salad

Serves 4 as a complete meal, 6 as an accompanying salad

¾ pound chunky fish (swordfish, tuna, tilapia, monkfish)

⅓ cup olive oil, for sautéing and for dressing

Salt and pepper, to taste

2 grapefruits (pink is prettiest)

½ pound rice, quinoa, or alternative-flour pasta (anything but spaghetti or linguine, as small shapes work best for pasta salads)

½ cup chopped red onion or scallion

2 tablespoons fresh oregano, or 1 tablespoon dried

2 tablespoons chopped flat-leaf parsley, cilantro, or basil

Stir-fry the fish in 2 tablespoons of oil in a skillet over medium-high heat about 4 minutes, until seared on all sides. Put in a large salad bowl and add salt and pepper to taste.

Peel and section grapefruits over the bowl to catch all of the juice; cut away all of the chewy membranes.

Cook the pasta until al dente (not mushy) and drain. Toss with a little of the olive oil so that it doesn't clump up while it is cooling to room temperature.

Add the pasta to the fish and fruit and add the remaining oil, onions, and herbs. Add more salt and pepper, if needed. Toss well and serve.

Asian Chicken Salad

Serves 4

1 pound boneless, skinless chicken breasts, cut in strips and stir-fried

¼ cup dark roasted sesame seed oil

¼ cup other salad oil (except olive)

⅔ cup orange juice (or canned mandarin orange juice)

2 tablespoons freshly squeezed lemon juice

Dash hot pepper sauce or oil

1 teaspoon grated, peeled fresh or frozen ginger

½ teaspoon salt or soy sauce (if it doesn't bother you)

1 cup tangerine, clementine, blood orange, or navel sections. (You can also use 1 can of mandarin oranges, using the juice instead of orange juice—see left)

4 cups Chinese (Napa) cabbage or romaine lettuce, shredded

1 cup roasted cashews

While the chicken is stir-frying, make the dressing. Combine sesame seed oil, salad oil, orange and lemon juice, hot pepper sauce, and ginger thoroughly with the salt or soy sauce. Pour ½ cup of dressing over the chicken in a bowl and toss well. Taste for seasoning.

Add the citrus fruit sections and toss.

Serve the chicken over shredded cabbage or lettuce divided on individual plates, drizzle the remaining dressing evenly over the plates, and top with the roasted nuts.

Tabouli with Quinoa

Serves 2–4

1 cup cooked Quinoa (see p. 294)

2 cups chopped parsley

¼ cup chopped fresh mint or 2–3 tablespoons dried (can use an opened tea bag)

½ cup chopped, peeled cucumber (or celery if cucumber doesn't agree with you)

1 large ripe tomato, chopped, or
1 cup cherry tomatoes, cut in half

2 scallions, chopped, or ¼ cup minced red onion

3 tablespoons freshly squeezed lemon juice

3 tablespoons salad oil

½ cup chopped, pitted green or black olives

Place all ingredients in a serving bowl and mix well. Let stand at least 30 minutes before serving.

Variations:

Use cooked grains other than quinoa.

For a complete meal, add pieces of cooked chicken or fish and serve in large lettuce leaves on individual plates.

Serve with stuffed grape leaves with Geoffrey's Tahini Vinaigrette (see p. 254) for a Middle Eastern–style meal.

Cold Sesame Noodles

Serves 3–4

1½ cups chopped, seeded cucumber or chopped celery

3 tablespoons freshly squeezed lemon juice

8 oz. 100% buckwheat Japanese soba noodles (or alternative-flour linguine)

6 tablespoons dark roasted sesame oil

1 tablespoon almond butter

3 tablespoons soy sauce, tamari, or shoyu, or use gomasio (salted sesame seeds) or salt to taste dissolved in vinegar

4 tablespoons rice vinegar or mirin (naturally sweet rice vinegar)

1 teaspoon or more grated, peeled fresh or frozen ginger

1 teaspoon or more minced garlic

1 bunch scallions, chopped

Hot pepper sauce or oil (optional)

Mix the chopped cucumber or celery and lemon juice to pour on top of finished noodles. Refrigerate.

Cook the noodles according to package instructions and rinse well or you might have a gelatinous, inedible mess. Put the noodles in a bowl and toss gently with a drizzle of sesame oil.

Mix the remaining ingredients, blending almond butter well. Pour the sauce over the noodles and mix well. Refrigerate.

Before serving, top with the cucumber or celery. This is a good summer Asian-style dish.

Salad Dressings

Salad dressings can also be used as marinade for poultry or fish or as sauce for cooked vegetables. Other recipes can easily be adapted using the oils of your choice, but here are some to get you started. Commercial dressings are usually full of fillers, so make some dressings and keep them in your fridge for up to two weeks.

Geoffrey's Tahini Vinaigrette

Makes about ¾ cup

½ cup oil

¼ cup rice vinegar or apple cider vinegar

1 clove garlic, chopped

½ medium-size shallot, chopped, or 1 tablespoon chopped chives

½ teaspoon sweetener, or stevia, to taste

Pinch salt

¼ fresh lime, juiced

Pinch cayenne or splash of pepper sauce

Blend all ingredients until smooth. Great accompaniment for a salad served with a spicy dinner.

Asian Dressing

Makes about 1 cup

½ cup dark roasted sesame oil

⅓ cup rice vinegar or mirin, naturally sweet rice wine vinegar

1 clove garlic, chopped

Dash soy sauce (tamari or shoyu), or pinch of salt if you are sensitive to soy sauce

Sweetener, to taste (omit if using mirin)

2 tablespoons sesame seeds, toasted

Blend all ingredients until smooth.

Avocado Cilantro

Makes about 1½ cups

½ cup peeled, pitted avocado

½ cup flaxseed or hemp seed oil

¼ cup balsamic vinegar, or apple cider vinegar with a touch of sweetener, to taste

½ cup fresh cilantro or parsley leaves

1 clove garlic

Salt and pepper, to taste

Place all ingredients in a blender or mash avocado in a bowl and whisk in other ingredients.

Tip: If making a Mexican meal, use ¼ cup fresh-squeezed lime juice instead of vinegar.

Lemon Vinaigrette

Makes about 1 cup

3 tablespoons freshly squeezed lemon juice

1 tablespoon wine vinegar

½ teaspoon salt

¼ teaspoon agave nectar or xylitol, or stevia, to taste

¼ teaspoon ground white pepper

¾ cup olive oil (olive oil is best in this recipe)

Mix all the ingredients except oil in a bowl or blender. Gradually whisk in the oil.

Summer Tomato Dressing

Makes about 1½ cups

1 small ripe tomato, quartered

1 clove garlic, peeled

¼–½ cup fresh basil leaves or other fresh herbs, washed and patted dry

½ cup olive oil

¼ cup balsamic vinegar

Salt and pepper, to taste

Process all ingredients in a blender until smooth.

Basic French Dressing

Makes 1½ cups

1 clove garlic, peeled

1 shallot, minced

¼ teaspoon salt

½ cup red wine vinegar or freshly squeezed lemon juice

1 teaspoon Dijon mustard

Salt and pepper, to taste

1 cup extra-virgin olive oil for classic flavor or as an alternative, hemp seed or flaxseed oil

Blend the ingredients, gradually adding oil. If you prefer less oil, you can use ½ cup oil and ½ cup vegetable or chicken broth.

Variations:

Add ⅓ cup mixed fresh herbs.

Add 1 teaspoon toasted cumin seed and use lime juice in place of lemon.

Add 2 tablespoons fennel seed.

Add 1 tablespoon chopped, rinsed capers.

Add ½ cup soaked sun-dried tomatoes and/or pitted olives.

If you eliminate the mustard and use a little fruit juice in place of vinegar and lemon juice, add poppy seed and a little sweetener.

Keep the mustard and add agave nectar, xylitol, or stevia for a honey mustard–style dressing.

Vegetables

Boil, broil, grill, steam, stir-fry, or roast—any way you prepare them, enjoy your vegetables. They are very important for your recovery.

ROASTED VEGETABLES A–Z

A quick and delicious way to cook many types of vegetables, roasting enhances natural flavors and brings out the sweetness. To roast, wash and spread vegetables out on a tray and drizzle with cooking oil (or salad dressing of your choice—see pp. 253–257 and then roast at 350°F about 20 minutes, or until soft but not soggy. Salt and pepper to taste.

Asparagus: Wash and cut off the woody ends.

Beans: If you can, eat fresh legumes. Trim stem ends from green or wax beans.

Bell peppers: Remove seeds and fleshy ribs from red, orange, yellow, and green peppers. Slice into thin strips.

Broccoli: Slice stalks in half or quarters.

Brussels sprouts: Cut into quarters (may take more than 20 minutes to roast).

Carrots: Baby carrots, slice lengthwise into halves; bigger carrots should be cut into quarters or eighths or small coins, depending on how large they are.

Eggplant: Cut into ¼-inch rounds, do not peel, but oil pan well.

Fennel: Cut off the end and, using only the bulbs, slice into ¼-inch rounds.

Leeks: Slice white part only in rounds or lengthwise into quarters.

Mushrooms: Use only the meaty kind. Slice big portobello mushrooms, or egg and chicks, or puff mushrooms into ¼-inch-thick slices; also slice button, chanterelles, or cremini mushrooms in half; or roast the very small ones whole.

Onions: Slice red, white, or yellow into ¼-inch-thick rounds.

Summer squash: Slice lengthwise into quarters.

Tomatoes: Roma or plum tomatoes work best; slice into ½-inch-thick rounds

Zucchini: Slice lengthwise into quarters.

Tip: The above-mentioned vegetables can also be roasted for 7 minutes and then grilled or broiled on all sides until done. If you wish, garnish with minced fresh herbs or minced garlic or sesame seeds. All vegetables can be steamed (place in steamer basket over boiling water). Denser vegetables like broccoli take 10-plus minutes, softer vegetables such as mushrooms, only 5.

Green Beans

Serves 4–6

2 pounds green beans, ends snipped and cut into 1-inch pieces

3 tablespoons olive oil

1 teaspoon lemon zest

1 tablespoon fresh rosemary, or 1 teaspoon dried

Prepare this recipe only if fresh legumes don't bother you.

Bring a large kettle of salted water to boil and drop the beans in to cook 5 minutes, until crisp but slightly tender. Drain.

While the beans are cooking, whisk together oil, zest, and rosemary in a saucepan over low heat. Transfer the beans to a serving dish and pour the warm sauce over.

Beets Julienne

Serves 4

3–4 large beets, baked or boiled and then peeled and cut into slices when cool

¼ cup chopped chives

¼ cup balsamic vinegar

⅛ cup olive, hemp seed, or flaxseed oil

1 tablespoon Dijon mustard

Salt and pepper, to taste

Place sliced beets in a serving bowl. Whisk together the remaining ingredients and pour over beets.

Red Cabbage, Sweet and Sour

Serves 4–6

1 yellow or white onion, sliced

1 apple, cored and sliced

2 tablespoons oil, for sautéing

1 medium-large red cabbage, cored and sliced into thin strips

3 tablespoons apple cider vinegar

2 tablespoons agave nectar or xylitol, or stevia, to taste

Water and up to 1 cup of apple juice or cider to cover vegetables and fruit

Salt, to taste

¼ teaspoon caraway seed (optional)

Sauté the onion and apple in oil in a heavy-bottomed saucepan or Dutch oven over medium heat. Add the red cabbage and barely cover with vinegar, sweetener, water, salt, and caraway seed. Simmer over low heat.

Do not let this burn or run out of cooking liquids, as burned cabbage is awfully smelly! You can use apple cider or apple juice in place of up to 1 cup of water; if you do, reduce the sweetener.

Tip: If you add a package of chopped turkey bacon or sliced chicken or turkey sausages during the last 15 minutes of cooking, you will have a complete meal to serve over rice or non-gluten noodles.

Cauliflower with Fresh Herbs and Garlic

Serves 4

1 medium-size head cauliflower, cut into florets

2 tablespoons olive oil

2 cloves garlic, minced

2–4 tablespoons chopped fresh cilantro, rosemary, dill, or parsley

Salt and pepper, to taste

Place florets in a single layer in a steamer basket over boiling water for 7–10 minutes. Heat the oil with garlic and fresh herbs in a small skillet until garlic is tender. Add salt and pepper to taste. Pour over cooked cauliflower in a serving bowl.

Celery Root Lasagna

Serves 2–4

2 celery roots, washed and peeled

Puttanesca Tomato Sauce (see p. 329) or any sugar-free tomato sauce

Slice root into ¼-inch-thick slices. Use as layers of "noodles" with sauce. Bake at 350°F for 30 minutes, until roots are soft and sauce is bubbly.

Eggplant *(only if you can handle this nightshade)*

Serves 3–4

Fried eggplant is delicious but it absorbs a lot of oil. It is healthier to steam the eggplant until soft, about 5 minutes. Eggplants can be peeled and cut into thin strips to make vegetable "noodles" for Puttanesca Tomato Sauce (see p. 329).

Ratatouille Provençale

Serves 4

1 yellow or white onion, sliced

1 large green bell pepper, seeded and cut into bite-size chunks

1 large red bell pepper, seeded and cut into bite-size chunks

3 tablespoons olive or other cooking oil

1 pound eggplant, peeled and cut into bite-size cubes

2–3 zucchini, cut into ¼-inch-thick rounds

6–8 plum tomatoes or 4–6 Roma tomatoes, chopped, or 1 (28 oz.) can whole plum tomatoes

4 cloves garlic, peeled and chopped

3 tablespoons plus ¼ cup fresh herbs: thyme, basil, oregano, parsley, chopped

1 bay leaf

Salt and pepper, to taste

Cook the onion and peppers in 2 tablespoons of oil in a heavy-bottomed saucepan or Dutch oven over medium heat until onions are translucent. Add the remaining tablespoon of oil, the eggplant, and zucchini. Cook, stirring frequently, at least 10 minutes.

As eggplant starts to stick to the bottom of the pan, add tomatoes, garlic, and 3 tablespoons of herbs. Stir. Reduce the heat to low, cover, and simmer until everything is tender.

Add bay leaf and salt and pepper, adjusting the seasonings to taste, and add the rest of the fresh herbs; basil is traditional, but any combination will do. Can also be served chilled with a garnish of lemon slice with each serving. Delicious over rice or other grain or noodles.

Emilia's Greens with Dried Cranberries

Serves 4

1 bunch Swiss chard or lacinata kale, or 2 bunches of well-washed spinach, washed and sliced

2 tablespoons oil

Salt, to taste

2 tablespoons balsamic vinegar or cooking sherry

2 tablespoons dried cranberries

¼ cup pine nuts (optional)

Do not drain the washed greens. Put the oil into a large pot over medium-high heat and stir in wet greens (greens start out big, then cook down as they wilt). Salt to taste and add vinegar and cranberries. Stir frequently. Add pine nuts, if you wish.

Greens as Lasagna Noodles

Serves 2–4

1 bunch large, leafy greens, washed and drained dry

Puttanesca Tomato Sauce (see p. 329)

Use 4 large leaves for each layer of "noodles" in a small rectangular lasagna pan with sauce.

Peppers, Sweet and Sour

(only if you can tolerate some sweetener) *Serves 4*

Sauce:

¼ cup tomato paste

¼ cup soy sauce (if tolerated), or 1½ teaspoons salt plus ¼ cup fruit juice

⅓ cup apple cider vinegar

⅛ cup of agave nectar or xylitol, or stevia, to taste

¾ cup water

1 tablespoon cornstarch or arrowroot

Peppers:

2 cloves garlic, minced

2 cups thinly sliced yellow or white onions

2 tablespoons cooking oil plus 1 tablespoon roasted sesame seed oil or 3 tablespoons vegetable oil

2 large red bell peppers, cut into thin strips

2 large green bell peppers, cut into thin strips

1 (15 oz.) can baby corn, or 2 cups frozen corn kernels (substitute 2 cups cooked carrots if corn is a trigger for you)

1½ cups raw or toasted cashews, whole or pieces

Stir the sauce ingredients together in a bowl and let stand. Meanwhile, sauté garlic and onions in oil in a wok or large skillet over medium-high heat. Stir-fry 3–4 minutes. Add pepper strips and continue cooking. Add a couple of tablespoons of water to prevent burning, if necessary.

Add the baby corn (or carrots) and cashews. Stir-fry 1 minute, then add the sauce mixture and simmer for 1 more minute, until the sauce thickens and bubbles. Stir until evenly thickened. Remove from heat and serve immediately over rice or cooked rice noodles.

Plantains Baked

Serves 2-4

Plantains are a starchy kind of banana. They are ripe when they are past yellow, almost turning black. Allow half a plantain per person as a filling starch. They are especially good with Mexican or South American dishes. Fry the green ones in oil, like chips (but they do absorb a lot of oil).

2 ripe plantains, skins washed and pricked with a sharp knife

Bake in a 400°F oven until the flesh is tender, about 45 minutes. Serve in its slit-open skin with a squeeze of flaxseed oil or hemp seed oil and a slice of lime on the side.

Potatoes for Breakfast, Lunch, or Dinner

Baked Potatoes (White or Sweet): Scrub, puncture with a fork, and bake in a 375°F oven 45 minutes or until soft. Eat hot with flaxseed oil or hemp seed oil, and salt and pepper to taste. Allow 1 potato per person.

Home Fries: Heat 3 tablespoons cooking oil in a skillet over medium-high heat. Thinly slice baked potatoes and fry about 15 minutes, flipping over halfway through. The hotter the oil, the crisper the crust, but the more fat you are ingesting. Salt to taste. Add a sliced shallot or onion and garlic, if desired. Allow 1 potato per person.

Mashed Potatoes: Use 2 medium-size potatoes per person. Wash, dice, and boil in salted water about 15 minutes, or until fork-tender. Mash until creamy, using olive oil instead of butter, and rice milk or nut milk. You can also boil 2 garlic cloves with the potatoes for additional flavor. Serve 1 cup mashed potatoes per person.

Fried Leftover Mashed Potatoes: Heat 2 tablespoons oil in a skillet over medium heat and fry mashed potatoes for 15 minutes.

Potato Pancakes for One: Hand grate 1 medium-size potato with a shallot or 2 tablespoons finely chopped onion. Add 1 teaspoon potato starch flour and ½ to ¾ teaspoon of Egg Replacer to thicken batter consistency. Fry in 1 tablespoon cooking oil, browning on both sides. Serve with applesauce.

Potato pancakes can be served with chicken or turkey sausage. While potatoes cook, place sausage on a tray in a toaster oven at 350°F for 15 minutes or fry in the skillet with the potatoes, browning on all sides.

Twice-Baked Potatoes

Serves 4

4 baking potatoes

1 yellow or white onion, diced

3 cups diced cooked vegetables; any combination, but mushrooms, broccoli, and carrots are a nice color combination

2 tablespoons cooking oil

¼ cup freshly chopped parsley and/or sage and basil, or 1 tablespoon dried

Salt and pepper, to taste

Chopped red onion or scallions, for garnish

Paprika (optional)

Scrub the potatoes and prick with a fork. Bake in a 375°F oven for 45 minutes, or until soft. Sauté the onion and vegetables in oil in a skillet about 15 minutes until soft. When the potatoes are done and cool enough to handle, cut each one in half and scoop out the flesh, leaving the skins intact for refilling.

Mash the potatoes together with herbs and cooked vegetables in a bowl. Add salt and pepper. Set the skins on a baking tray and mound in the filling. Bake at 350°F for 30 minutes.

Serve with chopped red onion or scallions and a dash of paprika on top, if desired.

Tip: Put in extra potatoes to bake so the next time this dish will only take about 40 minutes to make for another meal. Baked potatoes will keep in the fridge for several days.

Grilled Potatoes and Fennel

Serves 6–8

4 large Idaho potatoes, washed and sliced into ¼-inch slabs (lengthwise or crosswise)

2 large fennel bulbs, washed and sliced into ¼-inch rounds

Olive oil

Salt and pepper, to taste

1 cup Potato Garlic Mayonnaise (see p. 229), thinned with lemon juice to the consistency of cream

1 bunch scallions, chopped (optional)

Prepare the grill outside or preheat the broiler inside. Brush the vegetables with olive oil and season with salt and pepper. Cook the potatoes 2–3 minutes on each side. Cook the fennel about 2 minutes per side. Don't let them burn.

Arrange the vegetables on a platter and cover with the Potato Garlic Mayonnaise dressing. Garnish with scallions, if desired.

Rutabagas and Turnips

Serves 4

2 teaspoons salt

1 pound rutabagas or turnips, peeled and cut into 1-inch cubes

1 tablespoon olive, sunflower, or other allowed cooking oil

Pepper, to taste

Bring 2 quarts of water to boil, and add the salt. Add the vegetables and cook until soft, 15 minutes for rutabagas, 6–8 minutes for turnips.

Drain and mash. Add 1 tablespoon of oil and pepper to taste. These vegetables can also be mashed together with boiled potatoes, carrots, or celery root.

Roasted Root Vegetables

Potatoes, white or sweet

Celery root

Beets

Carrots

Jerusalem artichokes (sunchokes)

Leeks

Onions

Parsnips

Rutabaga

2 tablespoons olive, sunflower, or other allowed cooking oil

Salt, to taste

Wash, peel if necessary, and cut into bite-size chunks any or all of the vegetables listed.

Stir together in a large bowl with 2 tablespoons of oil and salt to taste. Place in a large casserole dish and bake in a 350°F oven for at least 1 hour. Stir from the bottom several times to prevent the potatoes from sticking.

Variation: For the last 15 minutes, add sprigs of fresh rosemary, walnuts, pecans, chopped broccoli, asparagus, or sliced chicken or turkey sausage.

Sautéed Yellow and Green Summer Squash

Yellow summer squash and/or zucchini
Oil, for sautéing
Salt and pepper, to taste
Pinch dried rosemary

Wash and slice squash into rounds. Sauté in cooking oil in a skillet over medium heat. Add salt, pepper, and rosemary.

Variation: Grate the squash and add salt. Place in a strainer and weight it down with a heavy plate or pan for about 2 hours. Squeeze out as much liquid as you can before sautéing in a skillet. The cooked squash will look like scrambled eggs. Great for breakfast with minced garlic, or wrapped in a corn tortilla covered with salsa.

Summer squash or zucchini can be sliced into thin strips and steamed to make vegetable "noodles." Steam over boiling water 5 minutes or until soft, but not mushy. Serve with Puttanesca Tomato Sauce (see p. 329). Allow 1 cup vegetables per person.

Baked Winter Squash

There are many kinds of squash to bake: acorn, butternut, Hubbard, pumpkin, and more. Split open squash, remove the seeds, and place in a casserole dish filled with 1 inch of water. Bake in a 350°F oven until flesh is soft, about 45 minutes. Winter squash makes a great starch alternative. Allow ½ cup to 1 cup cooked squash per person.

Tip: Winter squash is delicious plain, or with a little bit of hemp seed oil or flaxseed oil on each serving. The hollows can be filled before baking, either with a dip or spread (see pp. 225–230), or cooked grains moistened with 1 tablespoon of oil, or with chopped nuts and apple sweetened with a little sweetener of your choice and mixed with cinnamon and nutmeg.

Variation: Spaghetti squash is a hard winter squash with flesh that separates into strings when baked. Cook as above and serve with any pasta sauce (see pp. 227–228, 329–330).

Stuffed Pumpkin

Serves 4

1 small pumpkin

2–4 cups cooked rice, depending on size of pumpkin (see p. 295)

Oil of choice

2 teaspoons curry powder or mixed Indian spices

1 onion, chopped

1 green and/or red bell pepper, chopped

¼ cup diced dried apricot

¼ cup dried cranberries

½ cup pecans, walnuts, or slivered almonds

Preheat oven to 350°F. Cut off top of pumpkin by slicing around the stem end in a circle. Scoop out seeds and fibers.

Cook rice (see p. 295) in water or vegetable or chicken broth (left-over rice can be used).

Heat the oil in a large pan over medium heat and add curry powder or your own mix. Add the onion and peppers and stir-fry 5 minutes. Add chopped apricots, cranberries, and nuts to cooked vegetables until well mixed. Stir all ingredients together with rice in a large bowl.

Scoop rice mixture into pumpkin and place in a baking pan or casserole dish with a 2-inch depth of water. Bake about 45 minutes, until the shell is soft but not collapsing. This can be a great vegan contribution to a Thanksgiving feast!

Grains

Sensitivity to grains varies from one person to another, so make no assumptions and watch your reactions carefully. Even rice and corn can be troublesome to some people with MS, although these foods are the most likely to be tolerated, as is millet. Amaranth and quinoa (both high in proteins and other nutrients) are not technically grains but starchy seed fruits, and wild rice is only a distant cousin to regular rice, so they can add bulk and calories to your diet. Buckwheat or kasha also has no gluten. Kamut, spelt, and teff are more ancient grains with very low gluten and so are tolerated by many. According to the Celiac Foundation (celiac disease is an intolerance for gluten), oatmeal does not have gluten. Again, test your tolerance.

BREAKFAST GRAINS

Hot Cereals

The usual proportions for cooking whole grains are 2 cups of water to 1 cup of grain. If you are using ground flours to make hot cereal, as a rule use 3 parts water to 1 part flour.

Rice, amaranth, millet flour, or cornmeal hot cereal: Bring 1½ cups water and ½ cup flour or meal to a boil, whisking to avoid lumps. Add salt to taste. Reduce to low heat and stir until cooked to the right consistency, 5–7 minutes. Add more water if necessary. Serves 1.

Oatmeal (rolled oats, not steel cut, which take longer to cook): Bring 1 cup water to a boil and add ¾ cup rolled oats and salt to taste. Simmer over low heat for 10 minutes. Serves 1.

Variations: Cook a small amount of dried fruits with the grain—cranberries, raisins, chopped apricots, or prunes. If you do use dried fruit, avoid adding other sweeteners. Add ¼ teaspoon cinnamon and ½ teaspoon vanilla extract to add sweet flavor without glucose.

Serve with a squeeze of hemp seed oil or flaxseed oil, nuts, ground flaxseeds (nutty and full of omega 3 and omega 6), a tablespoon of nut butter, and/or rice or nut milk.

Tip: If you cook the cereal with no added sweet flavors, you can add leftovers to soups or stews to thicken them.

Fried Corn Grits

Serves 1

1 cup cooked cornmeal, left at least overnight in the fridge

3 teaspoons Egg Replacer (premixed egg substitute), or 2 tablespoons potato starch flour

2 tablespoons ground flaxseed

1 tablespoon cooking oil

Fruit-only jam for syrup

Mix the cornmeal, Egg Replacer, and flaxseed together. Heat the oil in a griddle or skillet over medium-high heat. When hot, drop silver-dollar-size spoonfuls in pan. Cook until a crust forms on the bottom, then flip carefully with a thin spatula to cook the other side. Serve with a small amount of fruit-only jam or jam thinned with water to make a fruit syrup.

Pancakes

Serves 2

3 teaspoons Egg Replacer

¼ cup potato starch flour

¼ cup white or brown rice flour

¼ cup cornmeal

¼ cup other alternative flour (amaranth, millet, spelt, buckwheat, chestnut)

2 tablespoons ground flaxseed

1 teaspoon baking powder

½ teaspoon baking soda

½ teaspoon salt

⅛ teaspoon cinnamon (optional)

⅓ cup sunflower seeds or chopped nuts

1 cup mashed banana, applesauce, and/or mashed sweet potato

1 teaspoon vanilla or almond extract

1½ cups nut or rice milk, plus additional if needed

Oil, for frying

Mix and whisk together the dry ingredients in a large bowl.

Mix the mashed banana with the flavoring extract and milk in a small bowl. Add to the dry indredients and stir until just blended. Add more milk if batter looks too stiff.

Heat the oil in a skillet or on a griddle over medium heat until a drop of water flicked on the surface spatters. Drop the batter by spoonfuls into the prepared pan and cook until bubbles show through from the bottom. The bottoms should be crisped and brown before flipping on the other side with a thin-bladed spatula. Keep the cakes small in diameter.

Add oil to the griddle surface as needed. Keep the first batches warm in a toaster oven on low heat until they are all done. Serve with agave nectar or with fruit-only jam or jam thinned with water to make a fruit syrup.

Buckwheat Pancakes

Serves 4

½ cup buckwheat flour

¾ cup mixed flours (rice, coconut, chestnut, spelt, amaranth)

¼ cup potato starch flour

3 teaspoons Egg Replacer

2 tablespoons ground flaxseed

1 teaspoon baking powder

1 teaspoon baking soda

½ teaspoon salt

1 tablespoon xylitol

⅓ cup sunflower seeds or chopped nuts

3 bananas, mashed, or 1½ cups (or more if batter appears too dry before adding milk) applesauce or mashed sweet potatoes

2 cups nut or rice milk, plus additional if needed

3 tablespoons sunflower seed oil

Whisk the dry ingredients together in a large bowl. Stir the wet ingredients together in a small bowl. Blend the wet ingredients into the dry and add milk if the batter looks too stiff—depending on whether you like thick or thin pancakes.

Heat some of the oil on a griddle over medium heat until a drop of water flicked on the surface spatters. Drop the batter by spoonfuls onto the griddle, and cook until bubbles appear on top, then flip over with a thin-bladed spatula. Add oil to the griddle as needed.

Tip: While the pancakes are cooking, keep the first batches warm in a toaster oven. Put ½ cup fresh or frozen fruit with 1 cup of agave nectar in a small saucepan and warm over low heat to make a great fruit syrup. Serve with a squeeze of hemp seed oil, flaxseed oil, or tahini instead of butter.

Berry Pecan Pancakes

Serves 4

½ cup spelt flour or mix of alternative soft flours (amaranth, millet, chestnut, coconut)

½ cup white rice flour

½ cup rolled oats

1 tablespoon baking powder

½ teaspoon salt

½ teaspoon cinnamon

1¾ cups rice or nut milk

1 tablespoon sunflower seed oil

1 cup fresh or thawed frozen berries (blueberries, strawberries, raspberries, or blackberries)

2 ripe bananas, sliced

½ cup pecans or other nuts or seeds

3 tablespoons sunflower seed oil

Whisk together the dry ingredients in a large bowl. Pour the milk and oil into a blender or use an egg beater to whip for 1 minute or until frothy. Pour the mixture into dry ingredients, mix well, and then stir in fruits and nuts.

Heat some of the oil on a griddle over medium heat until a drop of water flicked on the surface spatters. Drop the batter by spoonfuls onto the griddle and cook until bubbles appear on top, then flip pancakes over with a thin-bladed spatula. Add oil to the griddle as needed. Serve with fruit jams or syrups.

Granola

Serves 7–8

- 4 cups rolled oats
- ½ cup sesame seeds
- ½ cup sunflower seeds
- 1 cup ground flaxseed
- 1 cup chopped almonds
- ½ cup coarsely chopped walnuts or pecans
- ½ teaspoon cinnamon (optional)
- 2 teaspoons salt
- ⅓ cup sunflower seed oil
- ½ teaspoon vanilla or almond extract
- ½ cup agave nectar

Preheat oven to 350°F. Mix the dry ingredients in a large bowl. Mix together the oil, flavoring extract, and agave nectar in a small bowl. Pour the liquids over the dry ingredients and stir well to coat evenly.

Spread the mixture on a jelly roll pan (or any baking dish with shallow sides) and bake 30–45 minutes. Stir every 10 minutes after the first 15 minutes. Agave nectar can burn easily so turn the oven temperature down 5 degrees if it starts to burn and stir more often.

The granola is done when it is a nice golden brown color. Let cool completely before storing in an airtight container.

Walnut Quick Bread

Makes 1 loaf, about 10 slices

1 cup nut or rice milk

2 tablespoons sunflower seed or walnut oil

⅓ cup agave nectar

1 cup white rice flour

1 cup spelt flour, or ½ cup spelt and ½ cup mix of other soft flours (chestnut, coconut, etc.)

½ cup potato starch flour

1 tablespoon baking powder

1 teaspoon salt

½ cup ground flaxseed

1 cup chopped walnuts

Preheat oven to 350°F. Generously grease a loaf pan.

Combine the milk, oil, and agave nectar in a saucepan over low heat until blended.

Whisk together the dry ingredients, except the walnuts, in a large bowl. Gradually stir in the wet ingredients until well mixed and then stir in the walnuts. Turn the batter into the prepared pan and bake 1 hour, or until a wooden toothpick inserted in center comes out clean.

Let cool in the pan for 15 minutes, then turn out onto a wire rack to cool for at least an hour.

Corn Muffins

(Make these only if corn agrees with you.) *Makes 1 dozen muffins*

2 cups cornmeal

½ cup rice flour (white or brown)

1 tablespoon baking powder

¼ teaspoon salt

2 tablespoons ground flaxseed

3 tablespoons pepitas (pumpkin seeds)

⅓ cup xylitol, or ⅓ cup fruit juice and reduce milk to ⅔ plus ½ cup milk

⅓ cup sunflower seed oil

1⅔ cups rice or nut milk

Preheat oven to 375°F. Oil a muffin tin or line cups with paper liners.

Mix dry ingredients together in a large bowl and then add sweetener (or juice), oil, and milk in the middle and stir until smooth. This makes a wet batter. Spoon into the prepared muffin cups and bake until golden-brown, 15–20 minutes.

Variation: Use all cornmeal if you like, decrease xylitol to 3 tablespoons, and add ½ cup corn kernels. Use sunflower seeds instead of pepitas, or use different cooking oils.

Apple Almond Scones

Makes 1 dozen small scones

¼ cup spelt flour

¼ cup rice or other flour

3 teaspoons Egg Replacer

½ teaspoon cinnamon

½ teaspoon salt

¾ teaspoon baking powder

2 tablespoons xylitol

1 tablespoon ground flaxseed

⅓ cup grated apple (about half of a large apple)

1 tablespoon sunflower seed oil

4 tablespoons almond butter

½ teaspoon orange zest, or 2 sliced kumquats (optional)

Preheat oven to 350°F.

Mix together the dry ingredients in a bowl and whisk well. Place the grated apple into a bowl, add oil, mix well with almond butter, and add orange zest or kumquats, if using. Batter will be thick. Drop rounded tablespoons of batter onto a cookie sheet and bake about 10 minutes, until just browned on the bottom.

Richard's Banana Bread

Makes 1 loaf, about 10 slices

½ cup white or brown rice flour

½ cup spelt flour

¼ cup mix of other flours (chestnut, amaranth, millet, etc.)

¼ cup potato starch flour

¼ cup ground flaxseed

3 teaspoons Egg Replacer

½ cup xylitol

2 teaspoons baking powder

½ teaspoon baking soda

1 cup mashed bananas (about 3 bananas)

¼ cup sunflower seed oil

4 tablespoons nut or rice milk

¾ teaspoon vanilla extract

Preheat oven to 350°F. Oil a loaf pan.

Whisk together the dry ingredients in a large bowl. Mix the wet ingredients into a well in the center and mix well. Batter will be thick. Pour into the prepared pan. Bake 45 minutes, until a wooden pick inserted in the center comes out clean.

Let cool in pan 10 minutes, then turn out onto a wire rack to cool 50 minutes.

Ellen's Sourdough Spelt Bread

Makes 2 loaves

Although sourdough sometimes has a mystique about it and old starters that have been passed down through generations are prized, a starter is very easy to make and maintain. The process is one of mixing up some flour and water and letting it sit to ferment over a period of days until nice and bubbly. What it is doing is attracting the wild yeast from the air in your house. Interestingly, this process works better in old houses or ones where baking has gone on previously than in new houses. If you have trouble getting a starter going, you can add a small pinch of commercial yeast. Better yet, stir in a few whole organic grapes or berries. The chalky bloom on the skins will boost the process. Strain out the fruit after the starter is viable. Making sourdough bread is a longer process than regular yeasted bread, but results in a more flavorful loaf. This is due partly to the sourdough itself, but also to the time factor. A longer time frame allows the grain to develop maximum flavor so that even the simplest ingredients will yield superior bread without a lot of additions.

CREATING A STARTER

2 cups spelt flour

1½ cups water (no chlorine)

Grapes or berries or pinch of yeast (optional)

Choose a clear glass or plastic round container with a lid. (I use a 2-quart Rubbermaid.) It seems large, but there will be a lot of rising going on. Along the way, smell and taste your starter. It will have a sharp and tangy flavor.

Day 1: Measure into the container ⅔ cup spelt flour and ⅔ cup water. Stir vigorously and scrape down the sides with a spatula. Make a mark on the side of the container at the level of the mixture and let sit on the counter for twenty-four hours.

Day 2: The starter should have doubled in volume. Stir, add another ⅔ cup of spelt flour and ⅔ cup of water, and stir vigorously. Scrape down the sides and make another mark on the container. Let sit another 24 hours.

Day 3: Repeat the instructions for Day 2.

By Day 4 your starter should be ready to use. If you are not ready to bake yet, you can refrigerate the starter for up to three days.

MAKING THE BREAD

Sourdough starter	2 cups lukewarm water
6–8 cups spelt flour, or 4 cups spelt and 2–4 cups mixed other flours	1 tablespoon salt

The night before:

Take the starter from the fridge and stir it well. In the same container, add enough flour to make a fairly stiff dough. Scrape the sides and level it in the container. Put a mark on the side of the container and let sit overnight, 8 to 10 hours.

The next morning (time frame 5½ hours):

Notice the texture of the starter. It will be full of bubbles and should have doubled in volume at some point during the night, even if it is no longer that high.

Pour the lukewarm water into a large bowl. Measure out 16 oz. (2 cups) of the starter and add it to the water. Stir well, breaking up the mass of starter. It doesn't have to be perfectly blended. Add 1 cup of flour and stir well. Add the salt and stir again. Continue to add flour, ½ cup at a time, until the dough starts to hold together and pulls away from the sides of the bowl. Turn it out onto a lightly floured surface and knead, adding flour as necessary. Be careful not to add too much flour, as sourdough prefers to be on the moist rather than dry side. Knead for a total of 15 full minutes. To avoid adding too much flour, at some point during kneading you can switch from using flour during kneading to using water to moisten your hands to keep the dough from sticking, or if you have one, use a bench knife to keep scraping the board clean. The dough will become elastic and resilient. Place the dough into a clean, lightly oiled bowl. Turn dough to coat all sides with oil, cover the bowl with a damp towel or plastic, and set it away from drafts to rise for 2 hours. You can place it in your oven with just the oven light on. It should approximately double in volume.

Turn the dough out on your floured work surface and divide it into 2 equal parts. Knead each part briefly and form into 2 balls. Place on the lightly floured surface, cover with a towel, and let rest for 30 minutes.

Flatten each ball and roll up into a loaf shape. Place in oiled loaf pans. Press into the corners to flatten, then turn over so that the oiled surface is on the top and again press into the corners. Let rise, covered, for another 2 hours.

Preheat the oven to 450°F about 15 minutes before the end of the rising time. The dough should come up almost to the top of the loaf pans. Slash the tops of the loaves with a razor blade or very sharp serrated knife. Place the loaves in the oven. Spray the walls and floor of the oven with water and close the door to create steam. After 3 minutes, do it again. The introduction of steam helps to create a good crust. Bake 25 more minutes. The loaves are done when they look good and give a hollow sound when thumped on the bottom.

Cool the bread on a wire rack at least 20 minutes before slicing.

MAINTAINING THE STARTER

After you measured out the starter for the bread, there should still have been some starter left in the container. There doesn't need to be a lot. A tiny bit will do to colonize the next batch. To this bit, add 1 cup water and an equal amount of flour. Stir vigorously and scrape down the sides. This starter will be ready to use again in a couple of days, or refrigerate it up to a week or ten days. If you don't intend to bake so soon, once a week take the starter from the fridge and discard about 1 cup. Then add fresh flour and water in equal amounts to replace what you discarded. Stir well, scrape down, and put back in the fridge. You can even freeze it for longer periods. When you are ready to bake again, return the starter to room temperature and proceed from the instructions starting with the night before. Always smell your starter for that tangy sharp smell of a good starter. It is a living thing, and if well maintained can keep going a very long time. Sometimes, if neglected or contaminated by a different organism, the starter will die. You can tell by the smell. If this happens, discard it and begin a new starter.

GETTING MORE CREATIVE

Once you have mastered the basic sourdough recipe, you can get more creative. Instead of plain water you can use cooking water from vegetables; potato water is especially good. You can add nuts, seeds, or dried fruits, fresh or dried herbs, cooked leftover grains, or just about anything. Rosemary and pitted black olives are a great combination. Don't add more than 1 cup of other ingredients to the recipe, and add them only during the latter half of the kneading, incorporating them as you knead. You may have to adjust the amount of flour, depending on the moistness of the added ingredients. If you have a baking stone, you can experiment with free-form loaves on the stone, but I have found that spelt flour is softer and floppier than whole-wheat flour and benefits from the form of a loaf pan.

A FINAL WORD

The quantities given here are starting guidelines. Different batches of flour may absorb water differently. Even the humidity may have an effect. Trust your instincts. If the dough feels right, go with it. Bread is not as dependent on exactness as other types of baking are. The home bread baker does not have to guarantee a consistent product from batch to batch. It will always be good. So have fun and enjoy.

SOURDOUGH PIZZA

If you have leftover dough from breadmaking or want to make your own pizza, try one of these three recipes for sourdough pizza crusts.

Experimenting with these is essential to getting the kind of crust that you prefer for pizzas.

Suggested toppings for these pizzas: Puttanesca Sauce (p. 329), pesto, lightly sautéed onions, sliced garlic, minced mushrooms, sliced anchovies, chopped olives, chopped ground chicken or turkey.

Sourdough Pizza Crust 1

Makes 1 12–14-inch crust

½ cup spelt flour

½ cup chestnut, white rice, or other finely ground flour

¾ teaspoon baking soda

1 cup sourdough starter

2 teaspoons baking powder

½ teaspoon salt

¼–½ cup vegetable oil

Combine all the ingredients; mix well. Sprinkle the dough lightly with flour and spread in a pizza pan. Bake at 425°F for 10 minutes and remove from oven. Arrange toppings on crust and bake 10 more minutes until the (already cooked) topping is hot and bubbly.

Note: This makes one thick cakelike shortbread crust to be eaten with knife and fork. The main advantage is that you can use your fingers to form the crust in the pizza pan easily.

Sourdough Pizza Crust 2

Makes 1 12–14-inch crust

1 cup sourdough starter

1 tablespoon oil

1 teaspoon salt

1 cup spelt or mix of flours

Preheat oven to 425°F. Mix all the ingredients, working in flour until you have soft dough. Roll out flat. Sprinkle flour or cornmeal over the pizza pan and place dough on it. Bake about 10 minutes and remove from oven.

Put sauce and toppings on pizza, and bake until toppings are hot and bubbly. Consider using pesto instead of tomato sauce (see pp. 227–228).

Sourdough Pizza Crust 3

Makes 1 12–14-inch crust

Basic recipe for sourdough bread (see p. 284)

Preheat oven to 350°F. Add enough flour to the basic recipe to form a stiff dough. Knead 5–10 minutes.

Roll or stretch dough to fit greased pizza pans or cookie sheets sprinkled with cornmeal. Dough may be thick or thin, as desired.

Bake 10 minutes and remove from oven. Add toppings and return to bake 10 more minutes.

Note: The last two recipes make crisper, pick-up-to-eat crusts. However, all sourdough starter doesn't have the same rising power, so the results will vary. Experiment until you find the right texture and consistency for your tastes. Some people like crispy crusts (achieved best with a pizza stone heated in an oven 45 minutes to bake the pizza on) and some like them chewier. Nuts soaked 2 hours and then ground with oregano, salt, and/or Spike (a premixed seasoning) make a nice topping in place of cheese.

Burritos

Serves 1

These can be made for breakfast, lunch, or dinner. Corn and rice tortillas are sold in health food stores. Spread the center of a tortilla with ⅓ cup of cooked vegetables or protein salad (chicken, turkey, or tuna) made with Potato Garlic Mayonnaise (see p. 229). Roll up and heat in a toaster oven. Cover with salsa as desired.

DINNER GRAINS

Amaranth

Serves 4

1 cup amaranth

2 cups boiling water or broth

¼ teaspoon salt if using water

Place the amaranth and boiling water in the top of a double boiler over simmering hot water. Cover and keep checking for water absorption, as amaranth is very sticky. Add more water if necessary to ensure that amaranth is soft and thoroughly cooked.

Tip: Amaranth can be mixed with other grains like quinoa. Try ⅓ cup of amaranth with ⅔ cup of quinoa in 2 cups of boiling water in a regular saucepan. Cook 15–20 minutes.

Buckwheat Groats or Kasha

Serves 4

Kasha is roasted and has a deep flavor. Unroasted whole buckwheat groats, found in some health food stores, have a milder flavor. If you find it too strong on its own, combine kasha with white rice and cook just the same as rice.

1 small yellow or white onion or shallot, minced

2 tablespoons cooking oil

1 cup groats

2 cups broth

Salt, to taste

Cook the onion in 1 tablespoon of oil in a heavy-bottomed saucepan or skillet until just translucent. Add the remaining 1 tablespoon oil and the groats. Cook, stirring, about 3 minutes, until soft. Let stand 5 minutes. Add broth and bring to a boil. Cover and simmer about 15 minutes. Let stand, covered, 10 minutes. Salt to taste.

Kamut Berries Basic

Serves 3

½ cup kamut berries (or spelt berries)

Soak the berries overnight in cold water to cover by several inches.

In the morning, drain, if needed, and add to 4 cups boiling salted water. Lower heat, cover, and simmer about 30 minutes, or until tender but chewy.

This can be made into breakfast porridge or cooked with broth and used in any grain recipe.

Millet Risotto

Serves 4–6

1 tablespoon cooking oil

1 cup millet

3 cups hot broth

Millet is usually made with 2½ cups of water or broth per 1 cup millet. If you use 3 cups of liquid, it becomes even softer and more flavorful, like genuine risotto.

Heat the oil in a large saucepan or skillet and add the millet, stirring for 2 minutes. Add the hot broth, cover, and cook over low heat until all of the liquid is absorbed, about 35–40 minutes. Let stand, covered, 5 minutes.

Quinoa

Serves 4

1 cup quinoa (white or red)

2 cups salted water or broth

1 clove garlic

½ cup toasted seeds or nuts (optional)

Dry-roast the quinoa in a heavy-bottomed saucepan or skillet, stirring until roasted, about 3 minutes. Pour into a fine-meshed strainer and rinse well.

Pour the water or broth into a saucepan and add the wet quinoa. Add garlic. Simmer, covered, 20 minutes, or until all liquid is absorbed and each sphere is translucent, with the ring of germ apparent. Stir in seeds or nuts and let stand, covered, 5 minutes before serving.

Polenta

Serves 4–6

1 cup yellow cornmeal

4 cups cold water, or 2½ cups water and 1½ cups broth

3 tablespoons olive oil

1 small yellow or white onion, finely chopped

1 teaspoon salt

Mix the cornmeal with 1 cup of the cold water in a bowl; set aside.

Heat 2 tablespoons of the oil in a large saucepan over medium heat and cook the onion until translucent.

Bring the remaining water or water and broth to a boil and gradually stir in the cornmeal mixture. Reduce the heat to low and cook, stirring constantly, until the cornmeal is very thick and hard to stir. Add the onion. Sprinkle the salt over the top and stir in the remaining 1 tablespoon of olive oil.

Variation 1: Preheat oven to 350°F. Reduce boiling liquid to 1 cup water, 1 cup broth. Add 1½ cups of cornmeal mixed with 1 cup of water to the boiling liquids and stir for 15 minutes only. Grease a 2-quart baking dish and turn half of the polenta into the dish. Drizzle the surface with olive oil and fresh chopped herbs (oregano, parsley, basil, cilantro, etc.) and ½ cup of pine nuts or other chopped nuts or tomato sauce (see pg 329). Add the rest of the polenta to casserole, smoothing to cover. and pour ¼ cup of nut or rice milk or tomato sauce on top. Bake 35 minutes. Let stand 10 minutes before serving.

Variation 2 (Polenta Toast): Spread cooked polenta into a greased 9x13-inch baking pan and leave in the fridge overnight. Cut polenta into pieces and fry in oil in a skillet or on a griddle. Or, preheat the oven to 425°F, place cut polenta in a single layer on a greased cookie sheet, and toast on each side about 10 minutes. Serve with hot pizza toppings or any sauce and cooked veggies or meat or fish.

RICE AND OTHER GRAINS

All over the world, rice is eaten in its many colors—white, brown, black, yellow, and red. Health food stores often carry a variety in bulk so that you can buy small amounts and try them out for yourself. Short-grain brown rice has more nutritional value, as the nutrient-rich husk is left on, but white rice better absorbs flavors and sauces. If brown rice seems too "healthy" to you, try basmati brown rice, a long-grain rice that is lighter in texture. There are rice cookers to ensure that you get the finished product just right—not too sticky and not too dry. Here is a basic formula:

Brown, Black, or Red Rice

Serves 4

4 cups water

2 cups brown, black, or red rice

1 teaspoon salt

Bring the salted water to a rolling boil in a saucepan over high heat. Gradually pour in the rice, keeping the water boiling. Turn the heat down to medium-low (every stove is different, so experiment) and cover the pan. You don't want the rice to boil over, so lift the top quickly to reduce bubbles in the first 20 minutes—if that should happen, lower heat slightly, but otherwise keep top on until all the water is absorbed, usually about 45 minutes.

White Rice

Serves 2

1 cup rice

2 cups water

White rice cooks in less time than colored rice, from 20–25 minutes. Sushi rice is a very sticky variation for making sushi rolls (see p. 322).

Tip: Leftover plain cooked rice can be eaten as a breakfast cereal. Heat up with nut or rice milk, ½ teaspoon vanilla extract, and ½ teaspoon cinnamon in a small saucepan.

Risotto

Serves 4–6

1 tablespoon cooking oil

2 cups Arborio rice (short-grain white rice best suited for risotto) or medium-grain white rice

¼ cup white cooking wine (alcohol evaporates, leaving flavor behind) (optional)

4 cups heated broth

Heat the oil in a medium-size saucepan over medium heat. Add rice and cook, stirring, 1 minute, until rice is well coated. Add white wine, stirring until it is all absorbed.

Add broth a little at a time, just covering rice with a thin veil. Stir occasionally so that rice doesn't stick. Each time liquid is absorbed, add a little more. This should take 30 minutes; adjust heat accordingly so that the liquid absorbs over time.

Variations: Add lemon zest and sauté shallots, minced onion, or garlic in oil before adding rice.

Stir in other cooked vegetables 10 minutes before the end of cooking time.

Experiment with different flavors by using vegetable, chicken, or fish broth.

Wild Rice

Wild rice, not a true rice, is expensive but delicious and healthy. Used in stuffing recipes, it is often featured around Thanksgiving. There are packaged mixes of wild and other kinds of rice, which are less expensive and equally good. Follow the directions on the label.

Wild rice uses 3 cups of water to 1 cup of rice and 1 teaspoon salt to cook. Rinse wild rice well before cooking. Cooking time is usually 30–35 minutes. Let stand 10 minutes before serving.

Spelt Risotto

Serves 6

5 tablespoons olive oil

3 cups whole spelt soaked in cold water for 2 hours and drained

½ cup red cooking wine

10 cups stock simmering on low

Heat 3 tablespoons of the oil in a saucepan over medium heat. Stir in the spelt until the oil is absorbed. Add the wine and stir until absorbed, about 5 minutes total. Add a ladleful of stock to cover the spelt. Stir to keep spelt from sticking. Keep adding stock when it is absorbed by the spelt. Stir in the remaining 2 tablespoons olive oil to make the end product rich and creamy.

Teff

Serves 4

2 tablespoons cooking oil

1 cup teff

2½ cups boiling broth or water salted with 1 teaspoon salt

Teff, a tiny grain used in Ethiopia, is high in iron and fiber. Heat the oil in a large saucepan over medium heat. Stir in the teff and toast for 2 minutes, stirring constantly. Add the hot liquid. Cover and simmer over low heat 15 minutes, or until liquid is absorbed.

Variations: Stir cooked teff into other grains for a different flavor.

Cooked in 3 cups of water, 1 cup of teff can be eaten like morning porridge or spread like cornmeal into a pan and cut into pieces for baking or frying like polenta (see Polenta, p. 294).

Main Courses with Lean Protein

Lean protein is the other main pillar of the MS Recovery Diet, along with vegetables. Because it digests more slowly, protein keeps our hunger satisfied longer than vegetables alone. Though the usual sources of red meat have too much saturated fat, there are lower-fat alternatives like bison, elk, and deer. Some people might find themselves sensitive to the pork casings used in turkey and chicken sausages, which are suggested in a few of the recipes. If so, remove the casings and use the fillings only. More exotic game such as ostrich and emu are also very lean. For those of us who do not hunt, these can be found in some meat markets or can be ordered online. Wild game has the same amount of saturated fat as poultry, minus the skin, which is where the fat is stored.

Fish is an excellent source of protein, as it is rich in omega-3, but with the worldwide pollution of our oceans there is some concern about what else we are ingesting. The following lists of fish high and low in mercury should aid you in deciding what fish to choose:

Low-mercury: Anchovy, blue crab (mid-Atlantic), catfish, clams, cod (Pacific), flounder, haddock, herring, oysters (farmed), perch (ocean), plaice, pollack (Pacific), salmon (wild), sardines, scallops, shrimp, sole, tilapia (farmed), trout (farmed)

High-mercury: Blue crab (Gulf of Mexico), Chilean sea bass/Patagonian toothfish, cod (Atlantic), grouper, halibut, lobster, mackerel, mahimahi, orange roughy, oreo dory, oysters (eastern and Gulf of Mexico), pollack (Atlantic), shark, snapper, striped bass, swordfish, tuna

Fried Fish

Serves 2

½ cup cornmeal or rice flour

2 tablespoons ground flaxseed or other ground nuts or seeds

1 teaspoon salt

Pepper, to taste

2 teaspoons dried herbs: rosemary, oregano, dill, or premixed spices like lemon pepper, Cajun spices, or Spike

2 tablespoons cooking oil

2 thin fish fillets, about 8 oz. each (like trout, sole, flounder, tilapia)

Mix together the dry ingredients on a plate or flat-bottomed bowl.

Heat the oil in a skillet over medium-high heat. Rinse the fish and dip both sides of each fillet into the dry mix. Fry on both sides until flesh is cooked through and no longer translucent.

Baked Fish

These instructions are for thicker cuts. Cook fish 8–10 minutes per inch of thickness, or until internal temperature reaches 135°F–137°F (for tuna, usually eaten on the rare side, around 120°F).

Preheat oven to 350°F.

Marinate thick steaks or fillets (monkfish, cod, sea bass, red snapper, salmon) 3–4 hours or overnight in a mix of ⅔ oil and ⅓ lemon juice and salt or salad dressing to cover before cooking.

Bake in an ovenproof pan or dish 15–30 minutes, or until fish flesh is no longer translucent. Allow 8 oz. per serving.

Variations (before baking): Marinate fish in a mixture of dark roasted sesame oil, soy sauce (or salt), and orange juice to cover, with 1 teaspoon grated, peeled fresh or frozen ginger.

Sprinkle ⅓ cup chopped fresh herbs over fish: cilantro, rosemary, dill, marjoram, parsley, mint, etc. Or add ½ cup mixed chopped vegetables: red bell peppers, onions, shallots, garlic, tomatoes, mushrooms, pitted olives, etc. Or cover fish with lemon slices and 2 tablespoons rinsed capers.

Grill or broil thick steaks about 7 minutes per side. Prepare as instructed/suggested above.

Steam thick cuts in a fish steamer; a 2- to 3-pound piece should be steamed for about 10 minutes, depending on the thickness of the fish. Steam over 2 parts water mixed with 1 part white cooking wine to fill bottom of steamer, and place sprigs of fresh herbs on top.

Stuffed Fish

1 whole split trout (or other small split fish) per person, or 1 large split fish, ¾ pound per person

Preheat oven to 350°F. Wash fish and pat dry.

Stuff with spreads (pp. 225–230) or with any cooked grains seasoned with any salad dressing or dip. Use ¼ cup salad dressing or dip for each cup of cooked grain. Fill center of fish so that the two edges of the skin still meet, otherwise the filling will dry out.

Place in a greased baking dish. Bake about 30 minutes, or until flesh is no longer translucent and seems flaky.

Spicy Shrimp

Serves 2

1 onion, chopped

1 bell pepper, any color (red, orange, and yellow are sweeter than green), seeded and chopped

2 tablespoons cooking oil

1–2 cloves garlic, peeled and minced

12 plum tomatoes, chopped, or 1 (28 oz.) can whole plum tomatoes

1 pound fresh shrimp, peeled (fresh or frozen and defrosted), tail shells left on or removed, as desired

Hot pepper sauce

Salt, to taste

½ cup chopped fresh cilantro or parsley

Stir-fry onions and peppers in oil in a large skillet over medium-high heat about 5 minutes, until they start to soften. Add garlic and tomatoes and stir-fry 10 minutes, or until the tomatoes start to release their juices. Add shrimp when the vegetables are soft and cook about 3 minutes, until just turning pink. Overdone shrimp can become tough and chewy.

Add hot sauce and salt. Put in serving bowl or on individual plates of cooked rice and garnish with fresh herbs.

Tip: If you are using precooked shrimp, add at the end just to heat through.

Turkey Burgers with Shallots and Mushrooms *Serves 2*

2 tablespoons cooking oil

2 large shallots, peeled and sliced

8 oz. button mushrooms (or similar varieties), washed and sliced

¼ cup cooking sherry

1 pound ground turkey or chicken

Salt and pepper, to taste

Heat the oil in a large skillet over medium heat and stir-fry the shallots and mushrooms 5 minutes.

Add half of the sherry and continue cooking until vegetables are soft.

Form 4 turkey or chicken patties and place in pan one by one so they are completely flat on the bottom of the pan, pushing the vegetables aside. When they are halfway cooked (about 3 minutes), flip burgers over and salt and pepper the tops.

Add the remaining sherry and cook 3 more minutes, until the burgers are cooked through.

Variation: Italian patties are even more flavorful and use spices and milk-soaked bread, crackers, or cereal to flavor each burger. Then they are dipped in seasoned flour and fried as above.

Italian Meat Patties

1 cup sourdough spelt bread crumbs, or rice or corn crackers, cakes, or puffed cereal

1½ cups nut or rice milk (or enough to cover above grains in a small bowl)

1 pound ground turkey or chicken

3 teaspoons dried oregano, sage, rosemary, and/or thyme

2 tablespoons chopped parsley or cilantro

1 clove garlic, chopped

1 shallot or small onion, chopped

3 tablespoons soy sauce or Thai fish sauce, or 1 teaspoon salt

Pepper sauce, to taste

¾ cup any flour mixed with salt and pepper, to taste

2 tablespoons cooking sherry or red wine (optional)

Crumble the grain product into a small bowl and soak covered in nut or rice milk 2 hours. Squeeze out milk by hand.

Add soaked grain to ground turkey or chicken in a large bowl. Stir in dried and fresh herbs, garlic, shallot, and flavorings until combined. Form patties. If the mixture is too wet to hold together, add a little more puffed dry cereal or a few tablespoons of flour or Egg Replacer.

Mix the seasoned flour on a plate or in a shallow bowl. Dip the patties in the flour mixture on all sides and fry as above, with or without shallots and mushrooms. Simmering in sherry or red wine makes a delicious sauce, thickened by the flour coating on the burgers.

With added starch, makes 6 patties.

ASIAN STIR-FRY WITH CHICKEN AND VEGETABLES

Indian Style

Serves 4

2 tablespoons cooking oil

1 teaspoon ground turmeric

1 tablespoon brown or yellow mustard seed

1 tablespoon whole cumin seed

1 teaspoon asafoetida (optional, but enhances flavors)

1 teaspoon ground coriander

½ teaspoon cayenne

3 tablespoons grated, peeled fresh or frozen ginger

2 teaspoons salt

1 bunch broccoli, chopped

1 yellow or white onion, sliced

2 carrots, sliced

8 oz. snow peas

8 oz. mushrooms, sliced

1 (8 oz.) can water chestnuts, drained

1½ pounds boneless, skinless chicken (or turkey) breast, sliced into thin strips

2 tablespoons water or broth, if needed

Heat the oil in a large pot over medium heat and stir in spices and ginger. When the mustard seeds begin to pop, add the salt and the broccoli, onion, and carrots, and stir-fry 5–6 minutes.

Add the snow peas, mushrooms, water chestnuts, and chicken. Turn the heat down to medium-low and stir occasionally until all of ingredients are cooked through. Add 2 tablespoons of water or broth if necessary to keep ingredients from becoming too dry.

Serve with rice and with ½ cup fruit or a chutney of jam mixed with 1 tablespoon of vinegar.

Tip: You can substitute or add any kind of vegetables on hand—cauliflower, green beans, 1 small diced potato, parsnip, etc. If you don't have the above variety of Indian spices on hand, you can substitute 2–3 tablespoons of premixed curry powder, but it is fun to learn which flavors you especially love in curry by cooking them individually.

Mango Lhassi Drink

Indian meals can be spicy (although you control how much cayenne to add), so a cooling drink is often served. Pour into a blender canned light coconut milk and mango juice (or other tropical juice) in equal proportions. You can add 1 banana for thickness and garnish each glass with fresh mint, if available.

Thai Style

Serves 4

1 (13.5 oz.) can light coconut milk

3 stalks fresh lemongrass, or 3 tablespoons dried lemongrass (optional)

2 tablespoons peeled and grated fresh or frozen ginger or gangala root

1 teaspoon red pepper flakes (optional)

2 teaspoons salt

1 teaspoon ground turmeric

Juice of 2 limes

1 lime, sliced (for garnish)

1 bunch broccoli, chopped

1 yellow or white onion, sliced

2 carrots, sliced

8 oz. mushrooms, sliced

8 oz. snow peas

1 (8 oz.) can water chestnuts, drained

1½–2 pounds boneless, skinless chicken (or turkey) breast, sliced into thin strips

Hot cooked rice

½ cup chopped fresh cilantro

1 cup cashew nuts, toasted

You may substitute or add any kind of vegetables on hand—cauliflower, green beans, 1 small diced potato, parsnip, etc.

Heat the coconut milk in a large saucepan or Dutch oven over medium heat.

Meanwhile, peel off the dry skin of the lemongrass stalks. Use the blunt side of a chef's knife to gently smash and tenderize the soft part of the stalk.

Once the coconut milk is boiling, add the softened lemongrass and the ginger or gangala root. Turn the heat to low and simmer 15–20 minutes.

Remove the pan from the heat and strain the milk with a fine strainer. Add the pepper flakes, salt, turmeric, and lime juice to the strained milk. Return the pan to medium heat. Add the vegetables and chicken to the pan and cook 20–25 minutes, until the vegetables are slightly tender.

Serve with rice, small bowls of cilantro, cashews, and sliced limes for garnish.

Tip: This meal can be done in stages throughout the day. Prepare the coconut milk and let it stand while you cut and prepare denser vegetables. The cut vegetables can sit in the fridge, the milk can sit out covered while you rest. About 45 minutes before dinner, start the rice, cut up the meat and softer vegetables and add them with the denser vegetables to the coconut milk and cook. Toast cashews for 10 minutes on a tray in a 350°F oven, slice the limes, chop the cilantro, and rest again while the meal finishes cooking. You can keep the heat on very low beneath the vegetable/meat pot so it will remain warm if rice is still cooking.

Chinese Style

Serves 4

1 cup chicken broth

⅓ cup apple cider vinegar

1½ tablespoons cornstarch or arrowroot

Pinch sweetener, to taste

5 cloves garlic, chopped

1 tablespoon dark roasted sesame oil

1½–2 pounds of boneless, skinless chicken (or turkey) breast, sliced into thin strips

Soy sauce or salt, to taste

1 bunch broccoli, chopped

1 yellow or white onion, sliced

2 carrots, sliced

8 oz. snow peas

8 oz. shiitake mushrooms, fresh or dried, stems removed

1 (8 oz.) can of water chestnuts, drained

1 can baby corn, drained, if you can eat corn

1 can bamboo shoots, drained

1 head Chinese Napa cabbage, sliced

Hot cooked rice

Chopped scallions, for garnish

½ cup sesame seed, toasted (cook raw seed spread on a tray in 350°F oven 5 minutes), for garnish

You may substitute or add any kind of vegetables on hand—cauliflower, green beans, 1 small diced potato, parsnip, etc.

Whisk the chicken broth, vinegar, cornstarch or arrowroot, and sweetener together in a small bowl and set aside.

In a large skillet over medium heat, fry the chopped garlic in sesame oil until lightly browned. Add the chicken and soy sauce or salt and stir-fry over medium-high heat until the meat is crisp and browned. Add the reserved sauce and cook over high heat, stirring constantly, until the sauce is thickened and slightly reduced.

Turn down the heat to medium-low and add the fresh and canned vegetables. Simmer until the vegetables are barely tender.

Serve with rice, bowls of chopped scallions, and toasted sesame seeds as garnish.

Roast Chicken or Turkey

Estimate 1 pound per person when selecting poultry. Soak the bird in salt water or brine before you roast it (but not a self-basting bird, which comes already salted). Use a tall pasta pot, or if brining the Thanksgiving turkey, all 12 to 21-plus pounds of it, buy or borrow a large canning pot. For every gallon of water, use 1 cup of table salt, or see if you can buy sea salt in bulk at a health food store. The bird can soak four to six hours or overnight. Keep in a cool place if you can't store it in your fridge.

Rinse the bird inside and out, removing the giblets for cooking separately if you like. Seasoning the poultry on the skin surface, which you then discard because of too much fat, is not necessary. Use 1 cup of warm water to dissolve the salt, and then use cold water to just cover the bird. To the brine, add whatever herbs and spices you like: 1 to 6 tablespoons mixed sage, rosemary, thyme, pepper, and minced garlic, and up to 2 cups cooking wine in place of 1 cup water.

This method renders the meat very tender and flavorful without wasting herbs on the skin.

Roast Chicken

Preheat oven to 300°F. Rinse the chicken of brine water and fill cavity with 1 lemon (juices will be too bitter to make gravy), or 1 peeled orange, or 1 onion, 1 carrot, and 1 stalk of celery and/or sprigs of fresh herbs.

Turn the bird upside down on a rack in the roasting pan, with the breast and legs facing the bottom of the pan. This ensures that the juices will drip down into the breast, which you will turn right side up halfway through the cooking process to finish browning the top. Drizzle cooking oil all over the top surface and roast 1 hour at lower temperature for a small 4- to 7-pound chicken.

Flip over after 1 hour, and raise the oven temperature to 350°F. Roast 1–1½ hours, or until an instant-read thermometer inserted in the breast reaches 160°F–165°F, or in the fat of the thigh, not touching any bones, 170°F–175°F.

Roast Turkey

Preheat oven to 325°F. Rinse turkey of brine water.

Drizzle the top surface with oil, and add 1 cup of water to the roasting pan. Place a roasting rack on bottom of pan.

Roast upside down, filling cavity as above with 2 to 3 times the amounts listed for smaller bird, for 2 hours if turkey is under 18 pounds, or 2½ hours if up to 21 pounds. Flip it over and roast 60 to 90 more minutes, or until an instant-read thermometer tells you it is done. If the breast isn't brown enough, turn the oven up to 400°F for the last 10 to 15 minutes of roasting.

Barbecued Chicken Cutlets

Serves 3–4

2–2 ½ pounds boneless, skinless chicken or turkey breast

Barbecue sauce: (see p. 331)

Mix all of the sauce ingredients together. Marinate chicken for at least 4 hours in the fridge slathered with the sauce.

Grill outdoors, or broil in the oven 4–6 minutes per side, or bake as follows: Preheat oven to 300°F. Bake cutlets 1 hour. Turn up oven to 350°F, turn the chicken over, cover with sauce, and bake 30 more minutes.

Tip: This meat is delicious served with baked plantains, and sliced and fried onions and green or red peppers in 1 tablespoon of olive oil on medium-high heat. And/or make a salad and squeeze lime juice and drizzle salad oil on it.

Or toast some corn tortillas. Slice chicken into thin strips and assemble meat, salad, and cooked vegetables on top of tortillas to make tostadas. Serve with salsa and guacamole (see p. 229).

Or bake chicken at 300°F for 1 hour. Turn the chicken over. Top with sliced plantains, peppers, and onions tossed in 2 tablespoons olive oil and seasoned with salt to taste. Spoon the juices from cooking chicken and baste the vegetables. Turn up oven to 350°F and bake 30–45 minutes, or until everything is cooked through. Serve with a small bowl of chopped cilantro and lime wedges.

Chili with Turkey and Cashew "Beans"

Serves 3–4

2 tablespoons cooking oil

1 yellow or white onion, sliced

1 tablespoon chili powder, and/or hot sauce, to taste

½ teaspoon ground cumin

1 pound ground turkey or other ground meat

2 cloves garlic, minced

1 bell pepper, any color, sliced

1 small yellow squash or zucchini, sliced

8 plum tomatoes, diced, or 1 (28 oz.) can plum tomatoes, smashed with a spoon

1 cup cashews, soaked in water to cover 1 hour

1 tablespoon cocoa powder and 1 tablespoon sweetener, or to taste (optional)

Heat the oil in large saucepan or Dutch oven over medium-high heat and add onion and spices, stirring until onion is translucent. Add the ground meat, garlic, and other vegetables (except tomatoes). Cook, stirring, 5 minutes, or until the meat is halfway cooked through. Break up the meat and add tomatoes.

Drain the cashews and add to pot. Simmer over medium-low heat 1 hour. Add cocoa powder and sweetener if desired for a darker mole flavor. Tastes even better the next day. Serve with rice and salsa and salad with a guacamole and lime juice dressing or Geoffrey's Tahini Vinaigrette (see p. 254).

Shepherd's Pie

Serves 2–4

1 nut crumb or spelt piecrust (see p. 356)

2+ cups leftover mashed potatoes (see p. 267)

2 tablespoons cooking oil

1 large yellow or white onion, diced

1 large carrot, thinly sliced

½ cup sliced mushrooms

1 bunch Swiss chard or other greens, washed and sliced

½ cup ground chicken or turkey, cooked

1 tablespoon caraway seed (optional)

Gravy:

1 tablespoon oil

2 tablespoons flour or 1 tablespoon cornstarch or arrowroot

1 cup broth

Preheat oven to 350°F. Prepare crust.

Take leftover potatoes from fridge.

Sauté the onions and carrots in the oil in a skillet or Dutch oven over medium heat about 5 minutes. When onions are translucent, add the mushrooms and greens. Stir and cook 10 minutes, until greens are wilted. Add a little water if necessary. Add cooked meat and caraway seed and heat through.

Make the gravy by heating the oil in a small saucepan over medium-low heat. Add thickener to make a smooth paste. Add broth a small amount at a time, whisking constantly. If you are using flour, it will thicken after it comes to a slow boil. If you are using cornstarch or arrowroot, the gravy will thicken before coming to a boil, so be sure to remove it from the heat at that time.

Mound the vegetables and meat (whatever will fit) into the piecrust and pour the gravy over the top, distributing evenly. The mashed potatoes may need a little thinning with nut or rice milk before you smooth them over the top of the pie. Be sure to seal the potatoes right to the edge of the crust. Bake about 35 minutes, or until the potatoes are browned and the gravy is bubbling through.

Tip: This pie can be made with leftover cooked meats and vegetables. As long as you have enough to fill up the pie dish, use whatever you have on hand. Make sure you have enough mashed potatoes and gravy. Some health food stores sell premade gravy mixes, which are perfectly fine. Always check ingredients to make sure they don't contain food triggers.

Game Meat and Pepper Stew

Serves 4

2 pounds meat, cut into cubes (game cutlets such as elk, venison, or bison; or turkey or chicken breasts)

6 tablespoons cooking oil

Salt, to taste

⅔ cup chopped carrots

1 red bell pepper (or any color if red is not available), seeded and chopped

⅔ cup chopped leeks or onions (carefully washed and sliced)

⅔ cup chopped celery root (or celery if you cannot find the root)

2 cups inexpensive dark red cooking wine

3 cups chicken stock

⅓ cup tomato sauce or canned ground tomatoes

3 cups cubed butternut squash or pumpkin

4 tablespoons crushed peppercorns

Sauté the meat in 2 tablespoons of the oil in a sturdy casserole pot or Dutch oven over high heat. Brown all sides and add salt.

Transfer the meat to a bowl. Lower the heat and add 4 more tablespoons of oil to the pot. Sauté the vegetables, except squash, 2 minutes. Add the meat and sauté for 2 more minutes.

Add the wine, scraping up any browned bits on the bottom of the pan.

Continue cooking 5 more minutes, or until most of the wine is gone. Add the chicken stock and the tomato sauce and simmer 20 minutes.

Add one half of the squash and all of the peppercorns, making sure to add water if necessary to cover all of the ingredients. Cook over low heat 1 hour.

Check on the stew every now and then to make sure nothing is sticking to the bottom. Add the rest of the squash and simmer 20 more minutes. Salt to taste. This is delicious served over rice, diced boiled potatoes, or polenta (see polenta recipe, p. 294).

Turkey Provençale

Serves 6-8

3–4 pounds turkey breast (or other gamy dark meat like elk or venison)

⅓ cup olive oil

⅓ cup balsamic vinegar

⅓ cup red cooking wine or sherry

½ cup chopped dried apricots or Calimyrna figs

½ cup soaked sun-dried tomatoes

1 large onion or bottoms of 3 leeks, chopped

½ cup pitted green or black olives

4 tablespoons capers, rinsed

1 tablespoon fennel seed

1 tablespoon dried sage

1 tablespoon dried cooking lavender (essential)

1 teaspoon dried oregano

1 teaspoon dried rosemary

Salt and pepper, to taste

Chopped vegetables for roasting, amount depending on how much room your roaster has when the turkey breast is in it. Suggestions:

2–3 potatoes

2–3 carrots

1 large fennel bulb

2–4 plum tomatoes

Marinate the turkey breast the day before you roast it, in equal parts olive oil, balsamic vinegar, and red cooking wine or sherry. Make enough wet marinade to baste the turkey breast easily.

Combine the dried apricots or dried figs, sun-dried tomatoes, and onions or leeks and sprinkle over the turkey breast. Add olives, capers, the dried herbs, and salt and pepper. Flip the turkey over at least once in the morning so that both sides marinate.

The next evening or when ready to cook, preheat oven to 250°F.

Roast the turkey upside down 1 hour. Then flip the turkey so it is skin-side up and add as many chopped vegetables as the pan can accommodate. Drizzle with more oil and salt and balsamic vinegar and cooking wine if there are not sufficient juices to moisten the vegetables from the bottom of the pan.

Turn up the heat to 350°F and roast for 1 more hour, turning over vegetables once during that time, or until vegetables are soft and turkey is cooked through.

This is a good dinner to serve guests, as most of the assembling is done the day before, and the rest is cooking away while you sit down with your guests to appetizers and good conversation.

Italian Polenta and Ground Turkey

Serves 4

2 tablespoons cooking oil

1 yellow or white onion, chopped

2 fennel bulbs, chopped

2 stalks celery, chopped

1 red bell pepper, chopped

1 green bell pepper, chopped

8 oz. mushrooms, sliced

1 pound ground turkey or other meat

8 plum tomatoes, chopped, or 1 (28 oz.) can plum tomatoes or ground tomatoes or sugar-free tomato sauce

2 cloves garlic, minced

2 teaspoons dried oregano or 1 tablespoon fresh

Heat the oil in a large pot or Dutch oven over medium heat. Sauté all of the vegetables except tomatoes and garlic, stirring about 10 minutes, or until soft.

Add the ground meat, stirring to cook 5 more minutes. Add the tomatoes, garlic, and oregano. Cook 30 minutes, then simmer on low for at least 1 hour.

Homemade polenta and sauce can be made the day before, and taste even better if you do, so this is another good dinner to conserve energy for having guests (see polenta, p. 294).

Slice polenta into ½-inch-thick pieces and place on the bottom of a greased baking dish. Cover first layer of polenta with vegetable/meat sauce, then another layer of polenta and more sauce. Sprinkle with pine nuts or spread with a pesto (see pp. 227–228) before baking (optional, but great instead of cheese). Put in 350°F oven for about 30 minutes to heat until bubbling hot.

Pollet's Paella

Serves 4-6

There are many recipes for paella, which is a one-dish meal requiring a paella pot. It is traditional to use a ceramic one, but there are metal ones available as well. Paella usually combines fish, shellfish, and chicken (and sometimes sausage) with rice and vegetables. The trick to the best paella is the flavorful broth, which can be made earlier or the day before.

Broth

1 white fish or salmon fillet (a fish head, wrapped in cheesecloth for easy removal, is also great for this)

¼ cup white cooking wine

2 mussels

2 clams

1 onion, chopped

1 green bell pepper, seeded and chopped

¼ cup chopped fresh herbs: parsley, oregano, marjoram, thyme

2 cloves garlic, peeled

1 teaspoon salt

1 quart water, or to cover

Put all ingredients into a large saucepan or Dutch oven and simmer over low heat for 30 minutes, until fish is flaky and shellfish are open. Adjust seasonings to taste. Store in the fridge for several hours or overnight.

Paella

2 whole chicken breasts, cut into quarters, 2 whole chicken legs separated at second joint

4 chicken or turkey sausages, chopped (optional)

4 cloves garlic, minced

3 tablespoons olive oil

1 yellow or white onion, chopped

1 stalk celery, chopped

1 small fennel bulb, chopped

3 cups Arborio or other short-grain white rice

4 cups chicken broth

Pinch saffron (optional)

1 dozen cherrystone clams

1 dozen larger clams, whatever your fish store can order

1 dozen mussels

1 dozen fresh shrimp, size is up to your pocketbook, the larger the showier

Brown the chicken (and sausages if you use them) with the garlic in the olive oil in the paella pot over medium-high heat. Remove the meat to a plate.

Add the vegetables and sauté 5 minutes. Only add more oil if needed. Add the rice and stir until each grain is coated.

Push the ingredients aside and arrange the chicken and sausages so most of the meat is touching the bottom of the pot.

Pour in 2½ cups of fish broth and 2½ cups of chicken broth, add saffron, if desired, and arrange the shellfish on top. If pot is big enough, add ½ cup more of each broth after some has already been absorbed by the rice, about 30 minutes. Sometimes you may have to make a cover of aluminum foil to ensure rice is cooked through.

Check for smell of burning from the bottom of the pot. Lower heat and don't worry, keep it cooking—it will still taste great. Best of all, the whole assembly can be done in stages over the course of two days, and can cook on a simmering heat for about an hour until all the broth is absorbed and the clams and mussels on top are open and the shrimp is cy. All you have to do beforehand is keep an eye on adding if needed, and eat appetizers with your guests.

alad and you'll have a spectacular special dinner.

Comfort-Food Meat Loaf

Serves 4

1 pound ground chicken or turkey

½ cup puffed rice (or other allowed dry puffed cereal or crumbled muffins or cooked grain)

¼ cup chopped onion, or shallots, or chives

1 teaspoon dried oregano

¼ cup chopped parsley

¾ teaspoon salt

¼ teaspoon lemon pepper or regular pepper

3 teaspoons Egg Replacer mixed with 4 tablespoons of broth, or nut or rice milk or potato starch flour

2 tablespoons tomato paste (optional)

Preheat oven to 350°F. Mix all ingredients with hands until blended and pat into a small greased loaf pan. Spread with barbecue sauce (see p. 331). Bake 45 minutes.

Tip: Serve with garlic mashed potatoes (see pp. 267) and salad.

Kathi's Sushi Rolls

Sushi rolls can be made as appetizers for an Asian-style meal or served with fermented rice miso soup and cooked seaweed salad (check your local health food store or Asian grocery store) for a whole meal. If you can buy fresh sushi-grade fish, it is much the better. Sushi rolls make a great "sandwich" for taking to work or traveling, and have infinite variety for incorporating small amounts of leftovers and fresh vegetables. If your preference is to avoid raw fish, use cooked fish instead, so you can still enjoy these healthy and delicious wraps.

Basic ingredients

Toasted nori (large squares of a specific seaweed)

Cooked brown rice

Umeboshi paste or Asian Sunflower Seed Spread (see p. 226)

Green onion, sliced in quarters lengthwise

Avocado, peeled and thinly sliced

Variable ingredients

Lox, sliced

Sushi-grade ahi tuna, sliced in ½-inch strips

Canned fish steaks in chili oil

Pieces of cooked chicken or turkey

Carrots, shredded or julienne sliced

Cabbage, shredded

Shiitake mushrooms, sautéed in toasted sesame oil

Leftover cooked yams, mashed or sliced thinly

Cucumbers

Crushed nuts

Sesame seeds

Cilantro

Traditional sushi uses sticky white sushi rice with vinegar and mirin (naturally sweet Asian vinegar) for flavoring, but brown rice is also sticky and flavorful enough that you shouldn't need to add anything to it.

Nori is the seaweed that is used to wrap the sushi roll. You can buy it toasted or untoasted. If you buy it untoasted, be sure to toast it by holding it over a burner on your stove (either gas or electric will work) for a brief time until it begins to change color—from dark green to brownish. If you don't toast it, your sushi will be very chewy.

It helps to have a sushi mat, which looks like a small bamboo place mat. The mat is used to roll the nori around the ingredients and pack them in tightly. But you can make sushi without it—the rolls may just not be quite as tidy.

To assemble a roll: Place a slice of nori on a sushi mat or cutting board. Spread about ½ cup cooked brown rice in a 2-inch strip across the nori, near the middle. Leave about 2 inches on one side and 4 inches on the other.

Spread 1 teaspoon of umeboshi paste or Asian Sunflower Seed Spread on the 2-inch strip of nori.

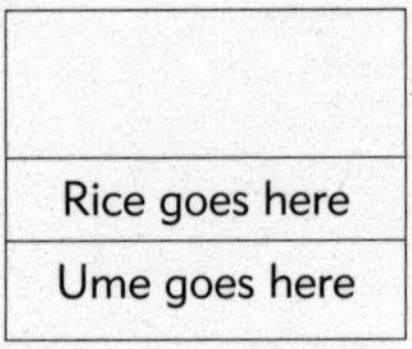

Rice goes here
Ume goes here

Place a couple strips of green onion along the edge of the rice nearest the umeboshi paste. Follow with a layer of the avocado slices (about ¼ of the avocado) and one or two other variable ingredients. Use a very small amount of each—just enough to ensure a little taste in each bite.

To roll the nori: Fold the edge with umeboshi paste over all the ingredients and then continue rolling. If you're using a sushi mat, you can lift the edge with the mat to control the foldover, tightening the pack before you continue rolling. As you roll, continue working the mat to tighten the roll.

To secure the roll, dab a little water on the dry edge of the nori just before you reach the end of the roll. The nori will then stick to itself when you finish rolling. Use the mat to tighten it one last time.

To cut the nori: Cut the roll in six equal pieces. Nori can be a little fragile to cut. Use a very sharp knife or a serrated knife and rinse it in water after every two to three cuts. Arrange with cut ends up on a plate.

Dipping sauces: Sushi is traditionally served with soy sauce. If you want to avoid soy, you can experiment with some other sauces and seasonings. For example, gomashio is a dry condiment that adds a salty flavor to food. You can buy it in health food stores, or make it very simply by toasting sesame seeds with salt in a pan on your stove and then crushing the seeds with a mortar and pestle. Sprinkle some on top of the sushi before you serve it, to achieve the traditional saltiness. But in truth, sushi tastes just great without any dipping sauce at all.

Sauces

From homemade tomato sauce to vegetable toppers, sauce can transform a plain supper of lean protein and vegetables into a gourmet meal with beauty and flavor.

Savory Cream Sauce *(without the cream)*

Makes 1 cup

- 1 tablespoon cooking oil
- 2 tablespoons flour, any kind
- 1 cup nut or rice milk
- Salt and pepper, to taste

Heat the oil in a small saucepan over low heat. Stir in the flour to make a smooth paste. Add milk, a few tablespoons at a time, stirring until it is all used. Salt and pepper to taste. The sauce will thicken as it comes to a slow boil.

Variations: Sauté shallot or garlic in the oil before adding flour. Add cornstarch or arrowroot mixed with a little of the milk, using a whisk to avoid having the sauce thicken at the bottom. Take off heat as soon as sauce thickens.

Or add 1 teaspoon dried herb or any savory spice, such as a pinch of saffron.

Or add ½ cup any seeds or nuts soaked (for an hour) and then ground up in food processor.

Brown Sauce

Makes 1½ cups

- 1 small onion, finely chopped
- 3 tablespoons cooking oil
- ¼ cup any whole-grain brown flour
- 1 cup vegetable or chicken broth
- Salt and pepper, to taste

Cook the onion in 2 tablespoons of the oil in a small saucepan over low heat 15 minutes, until brown, soft, and caramelized. Add another tablespoon of oil, and stir in the flour making a smooth paste. Add the broth, a few tablespoons at a time. Turn up heat to medium-low and stir until sauce begins to thicken. Season to taste. Add any spices as in prior recipe above.

Tahini Sauce

Makes 1 cup

This is a good, thick, hearty sauce to serve over starch and/or vegetables.

¾ cup warm water

½ cup tahini

1 clove garlic, minced

Juice of ½ fresh lemon

½ teaspoon curry powder or a mix of coriander and cumin if you have them (optional, but tasty for a Middle Eastern flavor)

Salt and pepper and a dash of Tabasco sauce, to taste

Whisk all ingredients together by hand or in a blender and serve.

Puttanesca Tomato Sauce

Makes enough for 1 pound of pasta

1 yellow or white onion, diced

1 bell pepper, any color, seeded and diced

3 tablespoons olive oil

1 teaspoon dried oregano

3 cloves garlic, minced

¼ cup red cooking wine

1 (28 oz.) can plum tomatoes, whole, ground, or diced

¼–½ cup olives, chopped, or 1 can chopped anchovies, drained and rinsed

1 (3.5 oz.) can tomato paste

Salt and pepper, to taste

Optional ingredients:

1 pound ground chicken or turkey

1 fennel bulb, diced

8 oz. mushrooms, chopped

1 zucchini, diced

1 yellow squash, diced

2 tablespoons capers, drained

¼ cup minced fresh herbs: parsley, cilantro, basil, oregano, thyme, marjoram

This kind of sauce is meant to be quick and tasty. The initial ingredients make it a very good sauce. If you have them on hand, the optional ingredients will make a great sauce.

Sauté the onion and pepper in the olive oil in a large saucepan or Dutch oven over medium heat until the onion turns translucent.

Add the oregano and the garlic, sautéing until the garlic is lightly browned. If you are using ground meat, brown for 3 minutes. If you are using fennel, add now and sauté 8 minutes, or until starting to soften. If you have the other less dense vegetables, add them and cook, stirring, for 5 more minutes.

Add the wine, tomatoes, and olives and stir to combine. Simmer 15 minutes and add as much tomato paste as needed to make the sauce the desired thickness. Add salt and pepper to taste.

Just before serving, add fresh herbs. Simmer on low for at least an hour to add flavor.

Barbecue Sauce

Makes enough for 2 or 3 boneless chicken breasts

½ (3.5 oz.) can tomato paste

1 tablespoon lemon juice

1 tablespoon apple cider vinegar

1 tablespoon olive oil

1 tablespoon dark sesame seed oil

1 teaspoon stone-ground mustard

1 teaspoon xylitol or agave nectar, or stevia, to taste

1 clove garlic, minced

½ teaspoon salt

½ teaspoon ground coriander

½ teaspoon ground allspice

1 teaspoon chili powder

Hot pepper sauce, to taste

Blend all ingredients. Use for any barbecue recipe (see chicken cutlet recipe, p. 313).

Vegetable Sauce

Serve over any grain, protein, and vegetable.

2 cups chopped vegetables

1 clove garlic, peeled and minced

½ medium onion, chopped

1½ cups water, or vegetable or chicken broth

½ teaspoon salt (optional; taste to see if broth is salty before adding any more salt)

¼ cup chopped fresh herbs, or 2 teaspoons dried

In a medium-size saucepan over medium-high heat, cook all ingredients together until the vegetables are soft. Remove from heat and cool.

Blend in a food processor or use a stick blender or a regular blender until sauce reaches smooth consistency.

Tip: Think of the color contrast to other foods you are serving. Suggested vegetables and herb combinations:

Carrots with dill, or with mint, or with 2 teaspoons grated, peeled fresh ginger (bright orange)
½ potatoes, ½ rutabagas with sage (pale orange)
Butternut squash with cinnamon (orange and sweet-flavored)
Asparagus and parsley, and 1 teaspoon lemon juice (green and delicate)
Onions with sage, rosemary, or thyme (white)
Beets with dill (purply red)
½ fennel, ½ onions, and oregano (pale green)
Red peppers and/or dill and oregano (red)
Green peppers, dill, oregano, and garlic (green)

Spicy Nut Sauce

Makes 1⅔ cups

1 cup nuts or mixed nuts and seeds, toasted and chopped

3 cloves garlic, chopped

3 tablespoons minced mixed fresh green herbs: cilantro, parsley, mint, and oregano are best

2 tablespoons balsamic vinegar

¼ teaspoon ground coriander

¼ teaspoon ground turmeric

¼ teaspoon ground fenugreek seeds (optional)

¾ cup vegetable or chicken broth

Salt, to taste

Hot pepper sauce, to taste

Pulse everything except the broth in a food processor several times, or until the nuts and seeds are finely ground with the garlic, herbs, and spices. Pour the mixture into a nonreactive glass or ceramic bowl and stir in the broth. Add salt and hot pepper sauce to taste. This sauce adds piquant flavor to just about everything. Cover and keep for up to 2 days in the fridge. Best served at room temperature.

Desserts

Judging by the American diet, we all crave not just fats, but also sugars, which can be very troublesome, not only to diabetics, but also to people with MS. There are sugar substitutes available, but many still have glucose, just lower amounts. Again, the watchword is to be careful and closely watch how your body reacts.

The following recipes will not be appropriate for everyone. If you are supersensitive to all things sweet, then do not experiment with these suggestions and recipes until your health, as noted by your symptoms, has stabilized to the point where you are willing to risk a temporary setback. Only you can judge between the benefit of satisfying a craving and experiencing an unwelcome symptom.

The following substitute sweeteners have been used in previous recipes in small amounts. For true desserts, they are used liberally, as sugar is in traditional baking. If you can tolerate the occasional splurge, then please enjoy and experiment substituting these three sweeteners in your own recipes. Use this cookbook as a template.

Stevia is sold as white or green drops or powder. It is made from a green leafy plant from South America. It is three hundred times sweeter than sugar.

Xylitol is made from both birch sap and corn. It is actually good for reducing the plaque on your teeth and is often used in toothpaste. It looks and tastes remarkably like sugar. It has a very low glycemic index and matches sugar in amounts for baking. Although the kind made from birch sap is less likely to give you trouble, some people do have digestive troubles with xylitol.

Agave nectar is sweet syrup made from the same cactus that is used to make tequila. It also has a low glycemic index. When using this in baking, you need to account for its liquid form by adding more dry ingredients. It can also burn at a lower temperature than sugar.

STARTING WITH FRUIT

Fruit has the most nutritional value when eaten raw. Cooking it will diminish some nutrients such as vitamin C. Here are some suggestions for optimal health value, with limited added glycemic content.

BERRIES

Berries have the lowest glycemic index of all fruit and are generally high in antioxidants. Enjoy a bowl of fresh berries in season. There are many kinds and they can be mixed for color and for sweet and tart combinations. Berries that are frozen straight from the field are also very good. You can buy them in season and freeze some yourself. Simply pick through, discarding overripe fruits, then rinse, drain, and spread intact fruit on cookie sheet and place in the freezer. When frozen, gather into a freezer bag and enjoy them thawed up to six months later.

FRUIT SALADS

The beauty of a fruit salad is that there are always different fruits to include each time you make one. Mixing them for color, texture, and flavor is an endless delight. Some possible special additions to a fruit salad:

Nuts and seeds, raw and toasted
Spice seeds such as fennel, anise, and coriander
Dried coconut
Avocado
Chopped mint leaves

Serve fruit salad in a bowl carved from large fruits such as melons and pineapples.

SLICED FRUIT

Along with the after dinner tea and coffee, put out a bowl of delectable washed fresh in-season fruit. This finish to a fine meal is made elegant by setting out a cutting board and sharp paring knives for each person. Put out your dessert plates and continue the dinner conversation as you slice off part of a fruit, peeling as you chat. Put the partially cut fruit back on the board and someone else will pick it up. In addition, set out a bowl of raw or toasted nuts and seeds. Have small towels or paper napkins handy for the juicier fruits. Offer a small bowl of water with floating flower petals on top to rinse the fingers along with the towels or napkins.

Variations: Serve small bowls of almond, cashew, or macadamia nut butters, or tahini with slices of crisp apples and pears. Use dessert plates and small knives for spreading.

Pineapple chunks, berries, grapes, banana pieces, and melons are all great for spearing with a wooden pick. Place a platter of these fruits in the center of the table, with a small dish of wooden picks.

FRESH MANGO

Sweet fresh mangoes are in a class by themselves and deserve status as a singular dessert. Slice the mango the long way beside the large flat pit inside. Cut the other half away from the pit. Use a sharp paring knife to skin the rim of fruit around the pit and slice away the pieces of fruit clinging to it. Save the pit for someone to chew on, like licking the bowl after making frosting. Take the halves with the skin on and score the fruit with the tip of the knife in crosshatch squares. Don't cut through the skin. Now flip the mango halves inside out so the scored squares are sticking out. Place in bowls and pass the napkins.

FRUIT WITH EXTRA SWEETENING

Fruits can be baked, grilled, or broiled, or poached in light syrup.

Baking: Preheat oven to 325°F. Quarter or halve peaches, apricots, plums, figs, pineapples, bananas, apples, or pears (removing all cores) and bake with a mix of 1 teaspoon of fruit juice, 1 teaspoon of sunflower seed oil, and a squeeze of lemon juice drizzled over every fruit you bake. Desiccated unsweetened coconut (from a health food store) makes a nice topping on the tropical fruits.

Grilling: This method requires no additional sweetener, as the grilling naturally brings out the sugars in each fruit. When you fire up the grill for cooking meat or vegetables, consider skewering some like-size pieces of fruit to cook as well. Sugars burn easily, so keep an eye on the fruit while it grills.

Broiling: As in grilling, you must beware of the sugars in the fruits burning. Consider adding grapefruit to the above list, only they may need a little sweetening. Halve grapefruits and sprinkle each half with sweetener of your choice. Broil for a few minutes.

Poaching: Canned fruits are poached, which by definition means they are cooked gently in some liquids, in this case, usually in heavy syrup. You can poach fruit pieces in a saucepan over low heat in two inches of fruit juice additionally flavored with a teaspoon vanilla, almond, orange, or mint extract.

Alternative flavorings could include just about any brandy or liqueur or an excellent-quality balsamic vinegar—just a drop or two of this kind of vinegar will do. You can also flavor the juice with ¼ teaspoon of cinnamon or nutmeg.

Simmer gently for 30 minutes, never letting the juice boil away. Additional sweetener of your choice or a squeeze of lemon or lime juice can also brighten up a lackluster fruit flavor—always taste first.

Fruit Gelatin

Serves 2–4

4 tablespoons agar-agar (the gelatinous seaweed gelidium, an alternative to gelatin)

4 cups fruit juice

1 cup sliced fruit and/or nuts

Add agar-agar to the fruit juice in a saucepan over medium heat and bring to a boil. Reduce the heat and simmer 5 minutes, until all of the seaweed flakes are dissolved.

Stir in fruit and/or nuts and ladle into dessert bowls. Put in the fridge for about 1 hour to cool until firm.

Baked Apple

Serves 1

1 large baking apple, such as Rome, but even the smaller McIntosh are delicious baked

1 teaspoon sunflower seed oil

¼ teaspoon cinnamon

1 tablespoon almond butter

Optional: pecan or walnut pieces; a few raisins or other dried fruit; 1 teaspoon xylitol or agave nectar, or stevia, to taste

¼–½ cup apple cider, apple juice, or other fruit juice

2 tablespoons water

Preheat oven to 350°F. Core the baking apple and peel the skin off the very top ¼-inch circumference. Rub a little oil over the apple.

Fill the apple center with a combination of cinnamon, nut butter, and, if desired, pieces of dried fruits or nuts, and sweetener to taste. If you use agave nectar, drizzle it over the top; if you use xylitol, sprinkle it over the top.

Set the apple in a baking dish with ½ inch of apple cider or other juice diluted with the water. Bake about 45 minutes, until apple is completely soft (cooking time depends on size of apple).

Check during baking so that liquids don't completely evaporate and burn. Baste apple with juice whenever you check it.

SUDDEN SWEET TOOTH URGES— WHEN FRUIT WON'T DO

Dry puffed cereal makes a nice snack if you sprinkle cocoa or carob powder with xylitol or stevia over the cereal and add a little rice or nut milk and a splash of vanilla extract. It will do much to assuage your sweet tooth.

Smoothies of banana and carob or cocoa powder, fruit juice, and sweetener can also do the trick.

Chocolate Halvah Substitute

Makes 2½ tablespoons

Halvah is a Middle Eastern delight made of sesame paste and compressed into cakes. Sometimes it is made with chocolate. This recipe is not real halvah, but it tastes just as good.

In a small cup, mix 1 tablespoon tahini, 1 tablespoon cocoa or carob powder, and 1 tablespoon agave nectar, xylitol, or stevia to taste. Mash together and eat tiny nibbles on the tip of a teaspoon.

Apple or Pear Brown Betty

Serves 4–6

¾ cup rolled oat flakes or absorbent flour like spelt, chestnut, or amaranth

¾ cup ground seeds and nuts (about ⅔ cup before grinding)

3 tablespoons sunflower seed oil

3 tablespoons apple cider, juice, or other fruit juice

1 teaspoon ground cinnamon

¼ teaspoon ground nutmeg (with pears, use ½ teaspoon)

1 pound apples, cored and sliced (3 medium-size apples; different varieties gives good flavor and varying textures)

¾ cup xylitol or agave nectar

3 tablespoons freshly squeezed lemon juice

Preheat oven to 350°F.

Mix all ingredients except apples, sweetener, and lemon juice in a small bowl. Use your fingers to rub it all together if necessary.

Grease an 8-inch square baking dish or a 9-inch pie plate. Press a third of the mixed ingredients in the pan, then cover with half of the apple slices.

Cover the apples with half of the sweetener, then sprinkle with 1½ tablespoons of the lemon juice.

Add half of the remaining mixture, then the rest of the apples, topped by the remaining sweetener and lemon juice. Finally, spread the remaining mixture over the top. Cover with aluminum foil and bake 40 minutes, or until the apples are nearly tender when poked with a fork. Uncover, raise the oven temperature to 400°F, and bake 10 more minutes, or until the top is nicely browned.

Variation: Use pears instead of apples and double the amount of nutmeg.

SAUCES FOR FRUIT

Marion's Chocolate Mousse

Serves 4

This versatile goody can be thinned with extra rice or nut milk for a sauce, left thick like whipped cream or a pudding, used to frost a cake, or served frozen like chocolate ice cream. People need never know that something this good is made with avocados.

2 ripe avocados

3 tablespoons carob powder

3 tablespoons cocoa powder, or 6 tablespoons cocoa powder instead of carob powder

4–6 tablespoons xylitol or agave nectar, or stevia, to taste

1 tablespoon flaxseed oil or solidified (refrigerated) coconut oil

⅛–½ cup rice or nut milk

Peel avocados and place in a food processor with the remaining ingredients. Blend until smooth, adding milk until desired consistency is reached.

Tip: You can also turn this into a cold pie with fresh fruit. See nut-based piecrust (pp. 355–356). Press crust into pie pan and bake 10–12 minutes. Cool and fill with chocolate mousse, sliced strawberries (high in antioxidants), bananas, or other fruit. Spread the top with almond or cashew topping (see p. 344), using a rubber spatula. Refrigerate until dessert time.

Cashew or Almond White Topping

Makes 1½ cups

1 cup cashews or almonds, soaked in water for an hour, then drained

1 teaspoon vanilla or almond extract

2 tablespoons xylitol or agave nectar, or stevia, to taste

1 tablespoon cashew butter (for smoother texture if desired)

Place all the ingredients in a food processor and blend. Use as topping over mousse or fruit, or add to cooked hot cereal for breakfast.

Coconut Cream Sauce

Makes 1½ cups

1 tablespoon sunflower seed oil

2 tablespoons soft flour (if you have it, use 1½ tablespoons chestnut and ½ tablespoon coconut flour)

1 (13.5 oz.) can of light unsweetened coconut milk

1 teaspoon vanilla extract

2 tablespoons xylitol or agave nectar, or stevia, to taste

Pinch salt

Heat the oil in a small saucepan over low heat and add flour to make a smooth paste.

Add coconut milk, a little at a time, stirring all the while. After it reaches a low boil and starts to thicken, add vanilla, sweetener, and salt. Serve at room temperature over hot or cold fruit.

Variation: Turn into chocolate coconut cream sauce by adding 1 tablespoon of cocoa powder to the flour and adjust sweetener to taste.

Banana Ice Cream

Serves 2

Peel 2 bananas and freeze. Grind broken pieces of frozen fruit in a food processor, adding 1 teaspoon vanilla extract and a little rice or nut milk for the desired texture.

Variation: Roll peeled bananas in crushed nuts and/or seeds. If you like, add 1 teaspoon cocoa or carob powder to the nuts. Freeze solid. Eat by wrapping a paper towel around the end to hold.

Mango or Berry Ice Cream or Sorbet

Serves 4

1 banana

1 cup chopped mango (you can use frozen)

Juice of ½ fresh lemon

¼ cup light coconut milk or fruit juice

3 tablespoons xylitol or agave nectar, or stevia, to taste

Put all ingredients in a food processor and blend until smooth. Pour the mixture into an ice-cream maker and follow the manufacturer's directions. Or, pour into a food processor bowl fitted with the sharp blade and place in freezer. Blend once an hour for at least 4 hours, until frozen through.

This is best eaten at once; if kept in the freezer too long, the ice cream loses its smooth consistency and becomes hard and compact. If you must freeze it, scrape it out of the food processor bowl and put it in a small storage container.

Variations: Use strawberries or other fruit in place of mango. For a sorbet, use fruit juice in place of coconut milk.

Blood Orange Sorbet

Serves 4

1½ cups freshly squeezed blood orange juice (around a dozen oranges)

4 tablespoons xylitol

1 tablespoon agave nectar

Heat all the ingredients in a saucepan until warm, but do not boil. Let cool. Pour the mixture into an ice-cream maker and follow the manufacturer's directions. Or pour into a food processor bowl with the sharp blade in place and put in freezer. Blend in the food processor every hour as it is freezing, about 4-5 hours, depending on how cold your freezer is, until frozen.

Serve the sorbet over a mix of sectioned citrus fruits (grapefruits and navel oranges), including any leftover blood oranges. If the fruits are especially sour, sprinkle with a little xylitol.

COOKIES

Sesame Carob Cookies

Makes 1 dozen cookies

¼ cup spelt flour

¼ cup white rice flour

2 tablespoons xylitol

1 tablespoon carob powder or cocoa powder

¾ teaspoon baking powder

½ teaspoon salt

1½ teaspoons Egg Replacer

2 tablespoons water

1 tablespoon sunflower oil

3 tablespoons sesame tahini

Preheat oven to 350°F. Mix all of the dry ingredients in medium-size bowl. Stir in the water, oil, and tahini.

Have an ungreased cookie sheet ready.

Mix the dough with your hands and compress into balls, making 12 cookies. Flatten slightly on the sheet. Bake 10–12 minutes. Let cool completely before removing.

Carrot, Coconut, and Almond Cookies

Makes 16 cookies

⅓ cup spelt flour

⅓ cup white rice flour

1 teaspoon baking powder

½ teaspoon salt

½ teaspoon cinnamon

⅛ cup dried unsweetened coconut

¼ cup xylitol

½ cup grated carrot

½ cup almond butter

½ teaspoon vanilla extract

2 tablespoons sunflower seed oil

¼ cup nut or rice milk

2 kumquats, finely sliced, or
½ teaspoon orange zest

Preheat oven to 350°F.

Whisk together the dry ingredients in a large bowl. Stir together the liquids in small bowl. Mix the liquids into the dry ingredients and stir thoroughly.

Turn the dough into 16 small balls and press flat on a greased cookie sheet. Bake 10–12 minutes. Let cool completely before removing.

Banana Oatmeal Cookies

Makes 2 dozen cookies

¾ cup spelt flour

¼ cup potato starch flour

3 cups rolled oats

½ teaspoon salt

3 teaspoons Egg Replacer

2 teaspoons baking powder

¼ cup raisins (traditional, but optional)

2 bananas, mashed

¼ cup applesauce

½ cup agave nectar

2 tablespoons sunflower seed oil

Preheat oven to 350°F.

In a small bowl, whisk together all of the dry ingredients except the raisins. In a large mixing bowl, mash the bananas and the liquids together.

Add the dry ingredients to the liquids. Add raisins if desired. Drop by spoonfuls onto lightly greased cookie sheets.

Bake 12–15 minutes, until golden brown.

Flourless Almond Butter Cookies

Makes about 16 cookies

- 1 cup almond butter
- 1 cup xylitol
- 1½ teaspoons Egg Replacer
- 1 teaspoon baking soda
- ½ teaspoon alcohol-free vanilla extract

Preheat oven to 350°F.

Mix all the ingredients in a bowl, and spoon dough from a tablespoon onto a greased cookie sheet, 2 inches apart. Bake 12 minutes, until cookies are puffed, golden on bottom, and still soft to touch in the center. Cool 5 minutes on sheet before removing.

CAKES AND MUFFINS

Chocolate Cake

Serves 20

½ cup spelt flour

½ cup white rice flour or chestnut flour, or other mix of flours

¼ cup potato starch flour

1 cup xylitol

¼ cup ground flaxseed (flax meal)

3 teaspoons Egg Replacer

1 teaspoon baking powder

1 teaspoon baking soda

½ teaspoon salt

3 tablespoons cocoa powder

3 tablespoons carob powder (or 6 tablespoons carob powder instead of cocoa powder)

3 medium to large bananas (to reduce underlying banana taste, use 1 cup applesauce or mashed sweet potato, or 1 mashed banana with ¾ cup agave nectar instead of xylitol)

¼ cup sunflower seed oil

¼ cup almond butter

¼ cup nut or rice milk (enough to give the batter the right consistency, pouring smoothly but not runny)

¼ cup coarsely chopped pecans or other nuts—optional

Preheat oven to 350°F. Grease and flour a 9x13-inch baking pan or line it with waxed paper.

Mix all the dry ingredients in a large bowl with a wire whisk, until thoroughly combined, breaking any cocoa/carob lumps into powder. Mash the bananas and stir in the other liquids in another bowl until thoroughly combined. Add to the dry ingredients and stir together until well mixed.

Spread the mixture evenly into the prepared pan. Bake 40–45 minutes, until a wooden pick inserted comes out a little wet and the sides of the cake are pulling away from the pan. If you bake the cake too long, it will be dry and crumbly. Let cool in pan for at least 30 minutes before serving.

Frost the cake with either ground almond or cashew topping or fruit spread, or if you are really going for chocolate decadence, you can use chocolate mousse as frosting (see p. 343).

Lemon Poppy Seed Cake (Pudding)

Serves 9

½ cup white rice flour (or chestnut flour or other mix of flours, including a small amount of sweet coconut flour)

½ cup spelt flour

¼ cup potato starch flour (½ cup if using agave nectar)

½ cup poppy seed

3 teaspoons Egg Replacer

1 teaspoon baking powder

1 teaspoon baking soda

1 cup xylitol

3 bananas, mashed (2 if using agave nectar)

¾ cup fresh-squeezed lemon juice (about 6 lemons)

1½ teaspoons lemon zest, or grated lemon rind

¼ cup sunflower oil

¼ cup cashew butter

Preheat oven to 350°F. Grease an 8-inch square baking pan for pudding, or a 9-inch square baking pan for a more cakelike texture.

Mix all the ingredients and pour into prepared pan. Bake 35–40 minutes, until cake/pudding is fairly solid, not gooey.

Frost with cashew or almond topping (see p. 344) or sprinkle with lemon juice sweetened to taste.

Pumpkin Dessert Muffins

Makes 1 dozen muffins

1 cup water

10–12 chopped dates (high in fructose—use 1 cup of agave nectar instead and eliminate water if dates' glycemic content is too high for you)

1 can pumpkin or equivalent freshly cooked

½ cup sunflower oil

2 cups almond flour

½ cup millet flour or amaranth or other allowed flours

¾ cup tapioca flour

2½ teaspoons baking soda

½ teaspoon salt

2 tablespoons cinnamon

1 teaspoon nutmeg

½ teaspoon ground ginger

½ teaspoon ground cloves

½ cup nuts

Preheat oven to 400°F. Grease a muffin pan or line with paper liners; set aside.

In a measuring cup, combine water and chopped dates. Heat in a microwave or in a small saucepan over low heat. Mash the dates when heated and soft.

Mix the pumpkin, water, dates (or agave nectar and no water), and oil in a mixing bowl.

Mix all the dry ingredients in another bowl until combined.

Pour the liquids over the dry ingredients and stir until combined. Spoon the batter into the prepared muffin pan. Reduce over temperature to 350°F.

Bake 35 minutes. Let cool before removing from the pan.

Stovetop Rice Pudding

Serves 4

1 tablespoon sunflower seed oil

2 cups Arborio rice or other white rice

4 cups nut or rice milk

Pinch of salt

½ cup xylitol or agave nectar, or stevia to taste

Fresh strawberries or other fruits

Put oil in a medium-size saucepan on medium-low heat. Pour in rice and stir to coat well. Add the milk, and turn up the heat, watching carefully until it reaches a boil. Reduce to a simmer and stir occasionally for about 30 minutes, until milk is absorbed.

Remove from heat, add salt and sweetener, and stir until well mixed, breaking up any clumps of rice. If your body can handle the extra dried fruit, raisins are a traditional addition. Serve with fresh fruit on top.

Sticky Rice Loaf

Serves 6

Soak four to six hours in a separate bowl:

½ cup cashews

½ cup white basmati rice

⅔ cup nut, rice, or low-fat coconut milk

Cover and set aside. Bring just to a boil:

1 cup nut, rice, or low-fat coconut milk.

Add:

½ cup white basmati rice

and simmer 5 minutes. Watch carefully that it doesn't boil over. Remove from heat and let parboiled rice also soak four to six hours. Add both soaked rice and nuts to a food processor bowl fitted with a sharp blade and add:

1 teaspoon salt

½ teaspoon baking soda

1 teaspoon vanilla extract

½ teaspoon cinnamon

1–2 tablespoons sweetener, to taste

Grind completely. It should look like watery gruel.

Grease a small loaf pan with sunflower seed oil or use 6-oz. ceramic ramekins. Set oven to 350°F. Add to mixture:

¼ cup nuts or seeds

2 kumquats, minced, or ½ teaspoon orange zest

¼ cup raisins or chopped dried apricots

Pour the mixture into the prepared loaf pan or ramekins and bake 30–40 minutes in loaf pan, 25–30 minutes in ramekins. The loaf should puff up just like an egg mixture and will sink shortly after cooling.

Serve with hot or cold fruit sauce made of fresh or frozen strawberries or other fruit and a little sweetener to taste. For strawberry "shortcake," turn the loaf out on a dessert plate and split in half. This is a mild sweet, good for an Asian meal dessert or sliced from the loaf for breakfast. Can be made the previous day and will last 4–5 days in the fridge.

PIECRUSTS

8-inch Crumb Crust

⅔ cup mixed ground sunflower seeds and nuts

½ cup any kind of flour

½ teaspoon salt

2 tablespoons sunflower seed oil

1 tablespoon sweetener (for a sweet pie) or 1 tablespoon dried herbs (for a savory pie)

Mix all ingredients until combined and press mixture into an 8-inch pie plate. Refrigerate 10 minutes. Top with filling and cook according to directions of filling recipe. Or bake crust at 350°F for 10 minutes, until golden brown, and let cool for a fresh fruit pie or a cold mousse filling.

Nine-inch Rolled Crust

⅓ cup solidified coconut oil (it becomes hard in the fridge) in place of shortening (butter or Crisco)

1 cup spelt and/or other flours

½ teaspoon salt

1 tablespoon freshly squeezed lemon juice

3–5 tablespoons ice cold water

Cut in the coconut oil with the flour, and add salt, lemon juice, and water by spoonfuls until dough sticks together in a ball. Refrigerate at least 30 minutes before rolling out.

The coconut oil tastes like coconut, so you can use this only for sweet pies, not savory ones. Make half as much again for adding a lattice crust or consider using a crumble topping as for Apple Brown Betty (see p. 342).

10-inch Oat-and-Nut Crust

1 cup rolled oats (if you can eat them)

½ cup almonds or cashews

1 teaspoon cinnamon

Pinch sea salt

1 cup spelt, or kamut whole-grain flour

⅓ cup sunflower seed oil

¼ cup agave nectar

Preheat oven to 350°F. In a food processor, grind the oats, almonds, cinnamon, and salt to a fine texture. Mix with the flour. Add the oil and agave nectar and mix to form soft dough.

Press the dough into a greased and floured 10-inch pie plate and flute the edges, if desired.

Bake 25 minutes until golden colored. Let cool while preparing cold filling.

9-inch Spelt Crust

3 tablespoons oil

2 tablespoons cool water

¼ teaspoon sea salt (optional)

1 cup plus 2 tablespoons spelt flour

Whisk oil, water, and sea salt together in a bowl. Stir in the flour and mix until evenly moistened. Press into a 9-inch plate. Fill and bake as required for the filling, or bake the empty crust 12 minutes at 375°F and fill when cool.

Apple Pie

Serves 6–8

6–8 apples, peeled and sliced (McIntosh are great for pies, but mixing varieties adds flavor and texture)

2 tablespoons sunflower seed oil

2 tablespoons apple cider or juice, if needed

1 teaspoon cinnamon

Pinch salt

½ cup xylitol or agave nectar

Sauté the apples in a heavy-bottomed pan with oil until softened slightly. Use cider or juice if apples are too slow in releasing their juices. Add cinnamon, salt, and xylitol or agave nectar, and simmer down until juices and sweetener achieve a syruplike thickness.

Put apples into unbaked pie shell and bake only about 30 minutes, as apples are already partially done.

Frozen Fruit Pie

Serves 6–8

20 oz. frozen fruit (berries, cherries)

1 tablespoon freshly squeezed lemon juice

½ cup xylitol or agave nectar

1¾ tablespoons cornstarch

½ teaspoon fruit liqueur (for cherry pie, use kirsch or almond extract)

Preheat oven to 350°F. Mix all ingredients together and let stand for 30 minutes, until fruit is melted and there is less of a cornstarch taste. Stir to coat well before pouring into an 8-inch piecrust. Bake 30–45 minutes.

Blackberry Pie

Serves 6

Crust

1 cup cornstarch

1 cup tapioca flour

⅔ cup garfava flour

⅓ cup sorghum flour

1 teaspoon salt

½ teaspoon xanthan gum

⅔ cup canola oil

⅓ cup agave nectar

Preheat oven to 400°F.

Combine the cornstarch, flours, salt, and xanthan gum in a bowl. Add the canola oil and mix well. This will be very moist—nothing like a "regular" piecrust. Add the agave nectar and mix with a large fork or pastry cutter. Mixture will now look more like a regular piecrust.

Divide the mixture into two parts, one a bit larger for the bottom crust, and refrigerate the remainder. Put the bottom crust in the middle of a pie plate, flatten, and push the crust out to the sides with your hands. When it looks like a regular crust and fills the pie plate, add the filling.

Filling

20 oz. frozen blackberries (2 bags)

3 tablespoons tapioca

⅓ cup agave nectar

Mix the berries, tapioca, and agave nectar and put the filling in the pie plate.

To make the top crust, take the remainder of the dough from the refrigerator and put on a piece of parchment paper. Flatten the ball of dough and continue pushing out toward the edges until you have a thin crust large enough to cover the pie. Invert the parchment paper over the filled pie and slowly peel off the parchment. Seal the edges of the pie, trimming excess, and slit top in quite a few places.

Turn oven down to 350°F and bake 45–50 minutes. Cool and serve.

Bibliography

Note: I have read extensively about MS over the past years and could not name all the sources of the information I've used, either from reading or from other people. The following list does include all the sources directly used and cited for this book.

Adler, Jerry, and Claudia Kalb. "An American Epidemic: Diabetes." *Newsweek*, September 4, 2000.

Austin, Phylis, Agatha Thrash, and Calvin Thrash. *Food Allergies Made Simple*. Sunfield, MI. Family Health Publications, 1985.

Barnett, Michael H., and Ian Sutton. "The Pathology of Multiple Sclerosis: A Paradigm Shift." *Current Opinion in Neurology*, 19 (2006): 242–247.

Bateson-Koch, Carolee. *Allergies: Disease in Disguise*. Burnaby, Canada: Alive Books, 1994.

Bland, Jeffrey. *Your Health Under Siege: Using Nutrition to Fight Back*. Brattleboro, VT: Stephen Greene Press, 1981.

Cantorna, Margherita. "Study Points to Positive Results from Vitamin D Supplements for MS Sufferers." Pennsylvania State University, 2001.

(This study was funded by the National Multiple Sclerosis Society.)

Chaudhuri, Abhijit and Peter O. Behan. "Multiple Sclerosis: Looking Beyond Autoimmunity." *Journal of the Royal Society of Medicine*, 98 (July 2005).

Compston, Alastair. "Making Progress on the Natural History of Multiple Sclerosis." *Brain*, 129, no. 3 (2006): 561–563.

Cook, Stuart D. *Handbook for Multiple Sclerosis*. New York: Marcel Dekker, 1996, 2001.

Cook, Stuart, D. "Multiple Sclerosis." *Archives of Neurology*, 55 (March 1998).

Cruveilhier, Jean. *Anatomie Pathologique du Corps Humain*. Paris: J. B. Bailliere, 1829–1842.

Dana, Charles, Smith Ely Jelliffe, et. al. *Multiple Sclerosis (Disseminated Sclerosis)*. New York: Paul B. Hoeber, 1922.

Embry, Ashton. Essays on multiple sclerosis, found at www.Direct-MS.org, 1995–present. (Includes "Probable Cause and Best Bet Treatment" and "Vitamin D.")

Erasmus, Udo. *Fats That Heal, Fats That Kill*. Burnaby, Canada: Alive Books, 1986.

Field, E. J. *Multiple Sclerosis: A Critical Conspectus*. Baltimore: University Park Press, 1977.

Filippi, M., and Maria Assunta Rocca. "MRI Evidence for Multiple Sclerosis as a Diffuse Disease of the Central Nervous System." *Journal of Neurology*, 252 (Suppl 5) (November 2005): 16–24.

Finger, Stanley. "A Happy State of Mind." *Archives of Neurology*, February 1998.

Fontoura, Paulo, Lawrence Steinman, and Ariel Miller. "Emerging Therapeutic Targets in Multiple Sclerosis." *Current Opinion in Neurology*, 19 (2006): 260–266.

Freedman, D. Michael, Alavanja Mustafa, and C. R. Michael. "Mortality from MS and Exposure to Residential and Occupational Solar Radiation." *Occupational Environmental Medicine*. 57 (2000): 418–21.

Freedman, Mark S. "Disease-Modifying Drugs for Multiple Sclerosis:

Current and Future Aspects." *Expert Opinion in Pharmacotherapy,* 7 (Suppl. 1) (2006): S1–S9.

Frohman, E. M., et al. "Characterizing the Mechanisms of Progression in Multiple Sclerosis." *Archives of Neurology,* 62, no. 9 (September 2005).

Galland, Leopold. *Power Healing: Use the New Integrated Medicine to Cure Yourself.* New York: Random House, 1998.

Gillson, George, Jonathan V. Wright, et al. "Histamine in Multiple Sclerosis, Part Two: A Proposed Theoretical Basis for Its Use." *Alternative Medical Review,* 5, no. 3 (2000).

Goodin, Douglas. "The Use of MRI in the Diagnosis of Multiple Sclerosis." *The Lancet Neurology,* 5, no. 10 (October 2006): 808-809.

Graham, Judy. *Multiple Sclerosis: A Self-Help Guide to Its Management.* Rochester, VT: Healing Arts Press, 1989.

Griffith, H. Winter. *Vitamins: Herbs, Minerals and Supplements.* Cambridge, MA: Da Capo Lifelong Books, 1998.

Hickey, William F. "The Pathology of Multiple Sclerosis: A Historical Perspective." *Journal of Neuroimmunology,* 1999.

Hobson, Katherine. "Solving the MS Puzzle." *U.S. News & World Report,* October 2, 2003.

Jonez, Hinton D. *My Fight to Conquer Multiple Sclerosis.* New York: Julian Messner, 1952.

Kantarci, Orhun, and Dean Wingerchuk. "Epidemiology and Natural History of Multiple Sclerosis: New Insights." *Current Opinion in Neurology,* 19 (2006): 248–254.

Kappos, Ludwig, Kenneth Johnson, Jurg Kesselring, and Ernst Radu. *Multiple Sclerosis: Tissue Destruction and Repair.* London: Martin Dunitz, 2001.

Kermode, A. G., A. J. Thompson, et al. "Breakdown of the Blood Brain Barrier Precedes Symptoms and Other MRI Signs in New Lesions in MS." *Brain,* 113 (1990): 1477–1489.

King, Martha. "Immunology for the Rest of Us." *Inside MS,* Spring 2003.

Lipski, Elizabeth. *Leaky Gut Syndrome.* New Canaan, CT: Keats, 1998.

MacDougall, Roger. "Recovering from Multiple Sclerosis." *Prevention,* 1974.

———. "The Speculative Future." *Let's Live,* August 1978.

Matute, Carlos, and Fernando Perez-Cerda. "Multiple Sclerosis: Novel Perspectives on Newly Forming Lesions." *Trends in Neurosciences*, 28, no. 4 (April 2005): 173–175.

Millan, J. H. D. *Multiple Sclerosis: A Disease Acquired in Childhood*. Springfield, IL: Charles C. Thomas, 1971.

Minagar, Alireza. "Multiple Sclerosis: Current Knowledge and Future Directions." *Neurological Research*, 28 (April 2006): 227–229.

Multiple Sclerosis Resource Center. *MSRC Introductory Pack*. Stansted, England: Multiple Sclerosis Resource Center, 1997.

National Multiple Sclerosis Society. *Cognitive Function*. 2006.

Ogilvie, J. C. *Overcoming Multiple Sclerosis*. Albuquerque, NM: Roadrunners, 1976.

Perlmutter, David. *Brain Recovery—Powerful Therapy for Challenging Brain Disorders*. Naples, FL: Permutter Health Center, 2000.

Rosner, Louis J., and Shelley Ross. *Multiple Sclerosis*. New York: Simon & Schuster, 1992.

Rudick, Richard A., and Donald E. Goodkin. *Multiple Sclerosis Therapeutics*. London: Martin Dunitz, 1999.

Somerville, Robert, project ed. *The Medical Advisor: The Complete Guide to Alternative and Conventional Treatment*. Richmond, VA: Time-Life Books, 1996.

Swank, Roy Laver. "Are You in Trouble?" *Swank MS Clinic and Foundation Newsletter*, April 1999.

Swank, Roy Laver, and Barbara Brewer Dugan. *The Multiple Sclerosis Diet Book*. New York: Doubleday, 1977.

Swiderski, Richard M. *Multiple Sclerosis Through History and Human Life*. Jefferson, NC: McFarland, 1998.

Thornton, Allen E., and Naftali Raz. "Memory Impairment in Multiple Sclerosis: A Quantitative Review." *Neuropsychology*, vol. 11, no. 3 (1997): 357–366.

Wallace, Joanne M. "Multiple Sclerosis and the Blood Brain Barrier: A Novel Approach in Integrative Care." *International Journal of Integrative Medicine*, 1, no. 5 (September/October 1999).

Warren, Sharon, and Kenneth Warren. *Multiple Sclerosis*. Geneva: World Health Organization, 2001.

Weil, Andrew. *Eating Well for Optimum Health*. New York: Alfred A. Knopf, 2000.

Woltman, Henry, H. Houston Merritt, et al. *Association for Research in Nervous and Mental Diseases*. Baltimore: William and Wilkins, 1948.

Appendix A. Supplements

There is no clear-cut answer about what supplements to take or in what amount, or even whether to take supplements at all. Valid arguments are made for both taking and for not taking supplements.

It has been strongly argued that these chemicals—and remember that these substances, though natural, are still chemicals—don't have the same positive effect on the body when isolated and processed out of the context of food. We do not have a full understanding of the way the body uses these substances and their interactions within the live cells of food, and therefore we can't determine how effective these substances are in isolation.

On the other side of this question, it has been shown that with the depletion of our soils, food is not as nutritious as it once was. Therefore, the argument goes, we need to supplement our diets with these essential vitamins and minerals.

For MS and the MS Recovery Diet, no one answer or approach stands out. Swank recommended only a multivitamin; MacDougall had a complete regimen; the ARMS group in England advocates using no supplements. Again, it is up to the individual to determine what works best.

Following are descriptions of the various vitamins, minerals, oils, antioxidants, and other supplements that are thought to be beneficial to MS recovery. Included in the write-ups are the natural sources for these as well as the supplement names. This will help in planning a well-balanced diet, geared to recovery as well as giving information if the decision is to include supplements.

Oils

Oils contain the essential fatty acids necessary for health, especially the omega-3 and omega-6 fatty acids. These are critical for healing, reduction of inflammation, the nervous system—all functions important to MS recovery. The fatty acids are crucial ingredients to cell membranes and myelin as well as a healthy digestive system. Vitamin D is found in fish oil (omega-3). The essential fatty acids are needed by the body to manufacture the prostaglandins, which regulate the immune system; as such they are anti-inflammatory agents.

Cold-water fish, oily fish, and wild salmon are good sources of omega-3, as are ground-up flaxseeds, flaxseed oil, and evening primrose oil. Make sure the oils are fresh; keep refrigerated so they don't oxidize.

Suggested oils for supplementation are mainly those rich in omega-3, since our modern diet includes many omega-6 oils.

Vitamins

Vitamins are actually unrelated organic compounds, but what they have in common is that they are all essential nutrients for our health and growth. There are two categories of vitamins; water soluble (B complex and C), which wash through our systems daily, and fat soluble (A, D, E, and K), which stay in the body longer. Each vitamin serves multiple functions, and all are found in a variety of foods.

The vitamin B complex comprises eight different chemicals that often act together to regulate metabolism, enhance immune and nervous system functions, and promote cell growth and repair, all crucial to MS recovery. The specific B vitamins most helpful to MS recovery are:

B_1 (thiamine) ensures proper nerve conduction. It is found in protein-rich foods like whole grains, peas, beans, and lean pork.

B_2 (riboflavin) is essential in maintaining mucous membranes as in the digestive tract, preserves the integrity of the nervous system, as well as working in conjunction with other B vitamins. It also has antioxidant properties. It is found in protein-rich foods like tuna, liver, and green leafy vegetables.

B_3 (niacin) is involved in many vital body functions. It synthesizes hormones, maintains nerve cells and blood vessels, supports the digestive tract, and detoxifies certain drugs and chemicals. Niacin is found in most protein such as liver, poultry, lean meats, fish, nuts, and peanut butter. The body can also manufacture niacin from dairy foods.

B_6 (pyridoxine) supports the immune system and nerve conduction. It is found in lean meats, poultry, fish, whole grains, brown rice, nuts, and bananas. Deficiencies here are rare and usually found in people with other health problems, like lactose intolerance and celiac disease, which create problems in absorption. This is best remedied by taking a multivitamin because taking too little or too much can impair nerve function.

B_9 (folic acid), which aides in metabolism, maintains the nervous system and intestinal tract, and controls the growth and repair of all cells. It is found in liver, kidney, eggs, fish, nuts, green leafy vegetables, peas, and beans.

B_{12}, which stabilizes the immune system, is crucial to the maintenance of nerve tissue, and is important in the formation of myelin. It is only found in animal products such as liver, meat, fish, and dairy foods. As a supplement, B_{12} is usually administered as a shot or a sublingual (under the tongue) tablet, as it is not easily absorbed.

Vitamin C is a powerful antioxidant and immune system booster. It is found in citrus fruits, bell peppers, broccoli, tomatoes, green leafy vegetables, strawberries, and cantaloupes. It is best to eat vitamin C foods or replenish your vitamin C daily, as it works through the system very quickly. As previously noted, it is water-soluble.

The fat-soluble vitamins include the following:

Vitamin A (beta-carotene) is a powerful antioxidant as well as a support to the intestinal lining. It is found in orange and yellow vegetables and fruits, dark green leafy vegetables, dairy foods, and organ meats.

Vitamin D, best known for its importance to bones, also supports normal nerve function. Sunlight is our most common source, but it is also found in fish oil and dairy products.

Vitamin E serves two important functions for MS recovery; it is an antioxidant and it is important to the proper function of the immune system. Vegetable oils, nuts, dark green leafy vegetables, organ meats, and seafood all are good sources of vitamin E.

Minerals

Calcium, which is the most common mineral in the body, is best known for its role in teeth and bones. However it is also important for proper nerve transmission. It needs to be taken with vitamin D to be properly absorbed. It is found in dark green leafy vegetables, sardines, salmon, and almonds, as well as dairy foods.

Copper strengthens blood vessels and nerves as well as performing many other functions. It is found in seafood, organ meat, molasses, nuts, seeds, green leafy vegetables, black pepper, and cocoa. Incidentally, water that passes through copper piping also contains this nutrient.

Magnesium helps to insure absorption of calcium. It is found in fish, green leafy vegetables, nuts, seeds, and whole grains.

Manganese is an antioxidant among other functions. Food sources are brown rice, nuts, seeds, beans, whole grains, peas, bananas, and oranges.

Selenium is also an antioxidant, which is boosted by the presence of vitamin E, as well as being a support to the immune system. Lean meats, seafood, whole grains, asparagus, garlic, and mushrooms are good food sources.

Zinc is integral to many functions, including cell growth, aiding the liver in removing toxic substances, and supporting the immune system. It is also an anti-inflammatory agent. It is found in protein-rich foods like lean meats, peanuts, oysters, and other seafood.

Antioxidants

In normal body processes, specifically those in which oxygen reacts with other substances, a by-product is free radicals. These molecules then roam through the body, causing damage to other tissue. This is thought to cause aging and disease. Substances that detoxify these damaging forms of oxygen are called antioxidants, and they can be made by the body or found in foods.

Many of the antioxidants have already been discussed: vitamins A, E, C, B_2; and the minerals selenium, zinc, copper, and manganese. Other antioxidants include:

Bioflavonoids or phytochemicals (vitamin P) are found in most any food. There are four thousand such compounds most concentrated in brightly colored fruits and vegetables, but are also found in wine and tea.

L-cysteine is an amino acid which, with its high sulphur content, acts as an antioxidant. It is manufactured in the body from protein sources like meat and whole grains. It also assists in the manufacture of glutathione, which is thought to help process out pollutants.

Other Aids

Acidophilus and probiotic formula are beneficial bacteria that help and protect the digestive system. They are naturally found in yogurt, kefir, and fermented foods, and are thought to enhance the immune functions.

Enzymes are made in the pancreas to help in digestion. There are three categories—lipase, which breaks up fat; amylase, which changes carbohydrates to simple sugars; and protease, which aids in converting protein to amino acids. The enzymes found in live food, when ingested, help with digestion.

Lecithin and its component choline are an important structural part of cell walls and of myelin. They also contain fatty acids and are found in all animal and plant products, including cabbage, cauliflower, beans, eggs, meats, seeds, nuts, and soy. Supplements are usually derived from eggs or soy, both often triggers for MS symptoms.

Glutamine is essential to healthy digestion. In the body it converts to an amino acid, all of which are manufactured from a protein sources.

Herbs

There are many herbal supplements used around the world and in this country that may well be supportive for the variety of body systems affected by MS. Here are a few common ones that are possibilities to investigate.

Psyllium seed husks are a safe laxative that can be used indefinitely without harm. They come in caps or a ground powder that can be added to liquids.

Saint-John's-wort is recommended for depression. It can affect liver function and therefore interact with other medications, so be sure to check with your doctor before taking it.

Rhodiola rosea is suggested for boosting energy, increasing muscular endurance and overall stamina, mitigating depression, and helping with mental concentration. It is sold commercially as Rosavin.

Echinacea and goldenseal are both used as natural antibiotics and can be taken orally or used topically for infections.

Conclusion

Notice that there is a lot of commonality in the foods mentioned for the various vitamins and minerals, reflecting the Paleolithic diet. In some cases, foods that have been identified as triggers were listed, however, in each list were safe foods as well. In following the diet it is a good idea to make sure you have all the essential vitamins and minerals covered by eating a sufficient variety of fresh fruits and vegetables.

If you choose to take supplements, check the base that carries the nutrient. Sometimes it can be egg or soy, known triggers to many people. Supplements are just that, they are additions to augment the dietary intake; they do not substitute for a healthy diet.

Appendix B.
Resources

More Information

The best resources are found at the website address www.direct-MS.org, which has essays, scientific papers, links to other helpful sites, and recipes. There are extensive bibliographies and citations to research that give more information and support about treatment.

Resources for Ordering Special Foods

If you don't have access to health food stores, here are some phone numbers, addresses, and websites of brand manufacturers to contact in ordering some of the ingredients that are necessary substitutes for grains, oils, etc. If you search online, you will find many more to compare prices with.

Ancient Harvest, distributed by Quinoa Corporation (quinoa and quinoa products)
Quinoa Corporation
PO Box 279
Garden, CA 90248

Applegate Farms (organic poultry products, including hot dogs, turkey bacon, deli sliced meats)
866-587-5858
www.applegatefarms.com

Arrowhead Mills (many organic grain and nut products, including puffed rice, corn, and millet cereals)
800-434-4246
www.arrowheadmills.com

Barlean's (flaxseed oil)
www.barleans.com

Bob's Red Mill (many whole grains, including polenta and white rice flour)
www.bobsredmill.com

Eden Foods (many products, including nongluten pasta, organic apple cider vinegars)
www.edenfoods.com

Ener-G-Foods, Inc. (Egg Replacer, potato starch flour, Rice Mix)
800-331-5222

Madhava Honey (agave nectar)
agave@madhavahoney.com

Smart Sweet (birch-derived xylitol, among other sweeteners)
508-252-5294

Spectrum (many organic cold expeller pressed oils, including sunflower seed oil)
www.spectrumorganics.com

Tree of Life (many organic and specialty items like organic walnut oil and supplements)
www.treeoflife.com

You can go online and find many websites for gluten-free substitutes. I've never ordered from www.shopglutenfree.com, but it is one of many sites that offers such products for sale; you still have to scan for other ingredients that might compromise your health.

Bodywork

To find exercise classes, consult your local physicians or physical therapists. Below is a list of the types and disciplines of bodywork that could be beneficial in your recovery. Remember to advise your teacher or therapeutic professional of your health issues, for maximum safety and benefit. Swimming is safe if you are heat-compromised.

Alexander Technique: Offers a specific focused awareness on body posture. When properly aligned, your muscles achieve greater release and movements become more effortless. It is another wonderful method to become aware of your own postural habits and accommodations that need to be released as you recover. I only had a short series of sessions many years ago, but I still remember the tender support I was given with my MS body.

Feldenkrais: A method of reminding the nervous system of healthy movement patterns and reintegrating these patterns into the existing repertoire of body awareness. There are two types of treatment: hands-on, one-on-one functional integration; and body awareness in classes taught through verbal instructions by the instructor. I work with an instructor one-one-one and practice these simple movements every day in my usual workout.

Pilates: Uses focused exercises on a mat and on specialized equipment to strengthen and tone the body, particularly the core muscles around the abdomen. You can take private sessions or work in classes. I practice some of the mat work every day at home without the Pilates equipment.

Shiatsu: A hands-on bodywork that uses the Asian meridian system of acupuncture, using pressure instead of needles. Chi, or life force energy, circulates through the body along certain pathways, or meridians, and stimulating them in specific points of contact promotes healing. Acupuncture and shiatsu have a similar basis but are not the same.

Yoga: There are at least six different branches of this ancient discipline that involve concentration and specific postures and forms of breathing to open the body to prana, or life force energy. It loosens, stretches, and relaxes—and some forms of yoga also strengthens—the body and the mind. Usually, it is taught in classes. There are postures I still practice after learning them thirty years ago.

Appendix C. Alternative Treatments

Here are short personal descriptions of alternative explorations Judi has used to support her healing with MS:

Acupuncture: An ancient Chinese practice that involves opening up blocks in channels of energy called meridians located throughout the body. The major systems and organs are all connected along these meridians, and by putting extremely fine needles (they do not feel like a pin used for digging out a splinter at all) into specific points along these channels, energies for restoring your health are freed. Western doctors have been amazed while observing major surgeries performed with only acupuncture used as an anesthetic. There are M.D.s who also do acupuncture these days. This was the second exploration after my diagnosis.

Apitherapy: Over six months, I stung myself five hundred times. The active ingredient of bee venom is melittin, a powerful anti-inflammatory substance, which makes some sense, given MS is an inflammatory disease affecting the myelin. Another component of bee venom is adolapin, a natural painkiller. The science is there, and although amazing testimonials abound, it didn't do much for me. If you have a friend with a hive, however, it is free and only costs you your time and some pain. Interestingly, I worked with Charlie Mraz, the one who made this healing popular in the United States, and he stung me along what turned out to be the liver and gallbladder meridians from acupuncture.

Biogram therapy: Originated by Dr. Richard Johnson. It is a visualization technique that can have profound healing effects. Dr. Johnson himself experienced a near-death event when he swallowed some poisonous chemical. He brought himself back to complete health, when the only other known victims with this specific accidental poisoning had died. The mind influences the chemistry of our body. His work embodies this theory beautifully. I had interesting but not long-lasting results from this work.

Continuum: It is hard to describe any of these methods accurately in just a few sentences. Continuum is particularly difficult for me to describe, as it is such a deep work and uses so many techniques within it. Technically, it is not for healing per se; healing is a by-product of doing the work. Essentially, Continuum is based on the premise that we are beings born of the water, from the primordial ooze to our mother's wombs, and then we evolved to become terrestrial. Continuum uses the neuroscience showing that our brain consists of three parts: the oldest reptilian brain; the mammalian, or limbic, brain; and the neocortex. All three work in synchrony. By reimmersing ourselves in liquid mediums using breath, sound, and wave motions, we can reconnect with the limbic brain and encourage our neurons to create new pathways wherever there are impaired spots due to illness or trauma. I find this works not only in healing my body, and amplifies any other method I choose, including this diet recovery program, but also heals my soul.

Cranial sacral work: This was invented by John Upledger, an osteopath. The cranial sacral fluid has pulsations that can be felt by practitioners when they place their hands at the base of the skull and along the spinal column. Practitioners can feel the blockages in this fluid and help to reinstate a healthy pulse. I do this work only with a trained osteopath, a doctor of osteopathy (D.O.). In my opinion, weekend training seminars that teach this work are not sufficient to lend authority to this important form of treatment. Since all of the nerve branches along the spine communicate to all parts of the body, a good osteopath can help enormously to restore vitality to people with compromised immune systems.

Homeopathy: In the late 1700s, Samuel Hahnemann discovered that "like cures like," meaning that substances that produce similar symptoms can cure the original ailment. In traditional medicine, for instance, radiation causes cancer, but in measured doses, it can cure it as well. Homeopathic remedies contain minutely distilled amounts of various substances, plants, and minerals that serve to stimulate the body's own healing mechanisms. In the United States, it was the major method of healing until the AMA, among other institutions, came down on the practice in the 1800s. It is practiced widely all over the world; Prince Charles is a major proponent. Each treatment is specific to the individual, and there is no application of "One size fits all." I used homeopathy for all of my children's ailments and found it very helpful for them. For myself, except for flu, I found it less helpful.

Hyperbaric oxygen chambers: All pathogens thrive in a lack of oxygen. As we who have MS move less due to our restrictions, we are less and less oxygenated. All cells need oxygen to utilize nutrients and eliminate wastes at maximum efficiency. Hyperbaric chambers were invented for deep-sea divers with the bends, which results when they descend or ascend too quickly and oxygen in their bloodstream is replaced with carbon dioxide, creating painful pressure. It was discovered that many ailments were eased when people spent time in hyperbaric oxygen chambers, as carbon dioxide was forced out by pressurized oxygen seeping in. The chambers are now used in medical facilities for various applications, including wound healing for diabetics. In Germany, if you have a stroke, you may sue the hospital if you are not placed in a hyperbaric oxygen chamber within a reasonable amount of time to prevent cell death for proximate cells. The chambers have been studied and used for MS for many years in England, which is where I first found out about them. I came home and bought a portable one for my home/office and used it every day for five years. It helped enormously with certain muscle groups and functions, bladder control, for instance.

Jin shin jyutsu: A Japanese energy healing system that can be very subtle or very dramatic. For me, as I recover my body on this diet, I can sense stagnant pools of energy that are relieved by the practitioners of this system. It is definitely helping me as I am re-membering my body and ridding myself of old bad physical habits.

Meditation: There are many forms of meditation, within every religious practice, and many without any specific spiritual orientation at all. Hospitals have found that meditation practices help people with chronic pain cope better with their lives. Many Eastern cultures have developed a science of mind that is as rigorous as any of our medical practices. Essentially, meditation gives you methods to step back and see the big picture of your life, and not to get lost in the anxiety-producing minutia of our daily lives. It isn't about rising above your life with your head in the clouds; it is about seeing yourself clearly and turning toward yourself and facing life with greater clarity. I meditate regularly for about twenty minutes a day and whenever I wake up at night and can't go back to sleep.

Osteopathy: Osteopaths work with the structure of the body to promote health in the physiology of the body. If our musculoskeletal system is functioning well, then the body is free to stay healthy and promote wellness and aid recovery from ill health or postsurgical trauma. Osteopathic physicians can use allopathic medicines, surgery, or drugs, and usually manipulate the body to align the skeleton and encourage all systems of the body to cooperate. My current osteopath teaches me a lot about what she is doing, and why, so that I feel I am participating in my sessions. Once, she moved a rib back into place, and another time she worked with her hands on my head and my trigeminal headache disappeared. My grandmother used to take me to an osteopath whenever I was ill as a child. My daughter had a trauma at birth, and osteopathy helped her immediately afterward in realigning her skull, and then later while the sutures in her skull were still pliable. I highly recommend osteopathy if you can find someone good. My osteopath is also a physical therapist and a Pilates instructor.

Prayer: Praying presupposes the belief in Someone or Something that you are praying to. This is very personal to each person. I have come a long way from praying to God as a child to help me find a library book almost overdue (it was under my bed) to praying in a much more generic way to the underlying movement of life that is everywhere within and around me. Faith is very individual and there is no one right or wrong path, in my opinion. For many people, there is only one way, and that is the source of their faith in life.

Psychotherapy: Ann discusses how to find a psychotherapist who is right for you in the chapter on depression. I worked with psychotherapists myself for many years, and I have counseled many people as well. MS is obviously not the only form of suffering on this planet of ours, just one of many. Helping people to accept and embrace their lives, no matter their history, can be part of everyone's journey.

Radionics: This is based on the principle that we emanate or radiate waves that are related to health or disease. There are many different kinds of machines that measure these emanating waves, and then the machines are adjusted to radiate back into your body the counterwave forms to mediate the disturbed waves. People who are sensitive to such wavelengths can also "read" you from a distance and send back to you appropriate healing waves. I was helped a lot by radionics through a period when I was ridding myself of all the mercury fillings in my teeth. At that time, I also did chelation therapy, which is a transfusion process that helped speed the removal of mercury from my body. I immediately felt greater mental clarity.

Shamanic healing: These are different hands-on and ritualistic healing procedures from all over the world. I have learned a great deal about my narrow definition of my body and my identity through exploring each one, from a Yuwipi healing ceremony conducted by a medicine man descended from the medicine man who healed Crazy Horse, to holding prayer beads carved out of human skulls while chanting a mantra in Tibetan. I have met people who were cured from supposedly incurable diseases through working with these shamans, and although it was never my result, I was healed at perhaps deeper levels of my own rigid thinking of what I deemed to be the right way or the right result. Hands-on healers exist in many traditions, including Christian, Kabbalistic, and Buddhist.

Index

About the Authors

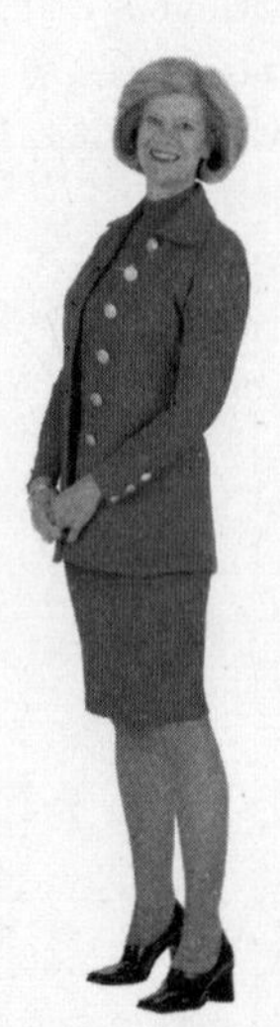

Ann D. Sawyer has been a psychotherapist and college instructor. Soon after her 1997 MS diagnosis, she was put on full disability. Since her recovery, she has pursued a new career as a novelist. Ann has also made it her mission to share the Recovery Diet and has been rewarded by seeing others recover from MS.

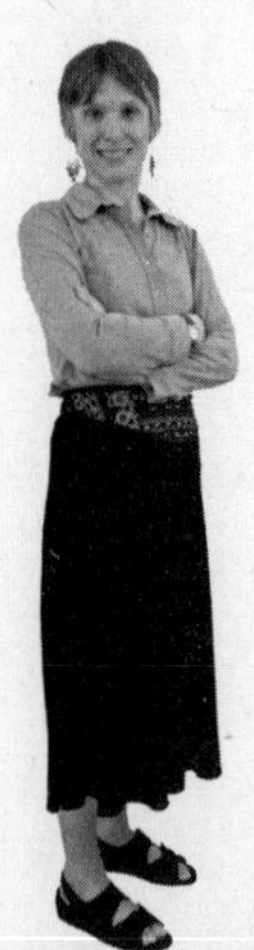

Judith E. Bachrach is a former dancer and movement instructor who has lived with MS for thirty-nine years. After trying numerous alternative therapies, as well as conventional drug therapy, with little success over the years, she began following the MS Recovery Diet in early 2006. Since then, her mobility, energy, and all functioning have improved dramatically.